Growing Up Healthy
the Next Generation Way

Growing Up Healthy
the Next Generation Way

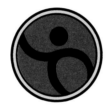

MARY ELLEN RENNA, M.D.

SelectBooks, Inc.

This book and accompanying DVD is meant as a source of information only. The information contained should by no means be meant as a substitute for the advice given your personal medical professional, who should always be consulted before beginning any new diet, exercise, or other health program.

All efforts have been made to ensure accuracy of the information contained in this book/DVD product as of the date of publication. The author and the publisher expressly disclaim responsibility for any adverse effects arising from the use or application of the information contained herein.

Growing Up Healthy, the Next Generation Way

This edition published by SelectBooks, Inc.
For information, address SelectBooks, Inc., New York, N.Y. 10003.

First Edition

ISBN-13: 1-978-1-59079-119-6
ISBN-10: 1-59079-119-3

Library of Congress Cataloging-in-Publication Data

Renna, Mary Ellen.
Growing up healthy, the next generation way / Mary Ellen Renna. -- 1st ed.
p. cm.
Includes bibliographical references.
ISBN-13: 978-1-59079-119-6 (pbk. : alk. paper)
ISBN-10: 1-59079-119-3
1. Health. 2. Physical fitness. I. Title.

RA776.R427 2007
613.7--dc22

2006102340

Manufactured in the United States of America

10 9 8 7 6 5 4 3 2 1

Food photography by Kenichi Sugihara

I would like to dedicate this book to my parents who gave me so much and asked for nothing, and to my husband Eric and children Sara, Spencer and Jamie who give this all meaning.

Contents

Foreword

People often look for shortcuts to staying healthy, looking fit and losing weight. The truth is that there are ***no shortcuts*** to maintaining optimal health, no magic meal plan that will take off the weight the way Photoshop® can. *Growing Up Healthy, the Next Generation Way* is not just another diet book with an exercise component thrown in. In fact, *Growing Up Healthy* is not about losing weight—it is about adopting a lifestyle that will help you and your family live longer and healthier lives. Part of being healthy is maintaining a moderate weight, and being overweight or obese is simply unhealthy. If you focus on your health by eating properly and exercising regularly, the likelihood is that you will lose weight if you are overweight. *Growing Up Healthy* will teach you about the only nutrition plan you will ever need. It outlines what every medical doctor and public health agency knows about good health. Its unique focus on children and their families will show you how to teach your children the good nutrition and exercise that will ensure generations of healthy children.

As a practicing pediatrician, most of what I do is to try and prevent disease before it occurs. I examine children every day and discuss the child's health with parents, who of course want to keep their children healthy and are always anxious to talk about my assessment. Obviously, it takes years of training to perform a physical exam and lots of experience to know when something is abnormal. But the majority of my time during a check-up revolves around issues of height and weight, nutrient intake and exercise routine.

Over the years, it became increasingly apparent that children were growing unhealthy and heavier. In fact, the incidence of obesity in children nationwide has increased nearly fourfold in the past thirty years![1] (SEE APPENDIX 1.) The two most important questions that I ask at virtually every check-up involve what the child is eating and what and how much exercise he or she is getting. The answers that I have received prompted me to document some solutions to a growing problem.

The current generation of children faces health challenges that were not an issue in prior generations. In spite of living in a land of plenty, many children are not getting proper nutrition; in addition, they are not getting sufficient exercise. It's a toxic combination, one that has produced a trend toward obesity and otherwise preventable diseases.

Part of my role as a doctor is to dispense advice. But one office visit, regardless of the value and wisdom of the advice given, cannot fix a lifetime of poor habits. Concerned with the growing obesity epidemic and frustrated by a limited means of contributing to the solution, I developed *Growing Up Healthy*. The program explains how ***healthy eating and exercise*** can improve the lives of children AND their families and shows how to accomplish this by providing a detailed, easy-to-follow plan. The plan is not a rigid prescription to be followed for a few months; it's a life plan designed to counter the unhealthy lifestyle that is the cause of not only overweight and obesity but also unnecessary disease and illness in our children.

The book discusses why 60 percent of Americans are overweight and why they are seemingly unable to reverse this dangerous trend. It also looks at why the overall health of children is declining and offers specific ways to thwart this epidemic. Understanding why children have become so unhealthy makes it easier to provide some solutions. The exercise DVD teaches children different types of exercises that are fun for the whole family and can be done at home without the use of fancy equipment.

My goal is to help children grow up to become healthy adults, but children need the help of their parents to achieve this goal. *Growing Up Healthy* is an important first step in improving the health of your entire family.

—MARY ELLEN RENNA, M.D., F.A.A.P., ABPNS
January, 2007

Introduction

Despite the medical advances of the 21st century, children all over the world now have more medical problems and shorter life spans than preceding generations.[1] (SEE APPENDIX 2.)

This may sound a little dramatic, but unfortunately it is true. There is now an overall decline in the health of the present generation of children in the U.S.[2] Why is this happening? We know that particular lifestyle habits are the cause of the problem and yet the health problems of the world are increasing instead of decreasing.[3] The rise of a more sedentary lifestyle combined with more reliance on convenience foods is causing an increase in preventable diseases worldwide. In fact, the incidence of obesity is growing faster in developing countries than it is in Western nations, where it is already an epidemic.[4] We are armed with the knowledge that eating better, limiting intake of red meat, decreasing fat and getting the proper amount of exercise can decrease the risk of developing heart disease and several other preventable diseases, yet we still continue to eat ourselves into poor health. Why are we unable to reverse this trend? *Growing Up Healthy* addresses this question and provides some solutions to the problem. The goal is to arm our children with the knowledge and skills needed to protect their health.

Certainly there are people who are not aware of this overall trend and its consequences. But even among those who are aware of it, many do not acknowledge that lifestyle, exercise and eating habits truly have an effect on diseases. In my practice, I am in daily contact with many parents who need to be convinced that if dramatic changes are not made in their child's habits, the child is likely to suffer from more diseases and have a shorter life expectancy than the parents. I also see many parents who believe that no changes are needed because their child does not have a weight problem. It is important to remember that not all children who have poor eating and exercise habits are overweight. This fact often lulls parents into a false sense of security; a child can be thin or muscular but if the child is not eating well and exercising, he or she will still be at risk.

Parents have their children's interests at heart and they naturally would do anything they could to help their children live longer and healthier lives. I believe our current health situation is so critical that once parents recognize the impact of their current habits on the long-term health of their children, they will make changes for themselves and serve as role models to guide their children.

Although this negative health trend is continuing, there are ways to solve the problem, and this is why I developed the Next Generation Fitness Program. We all need to improve ourselves in developing healthier lifestyles, and the younger you are, the easier this is to accomplish.[5] ***Children are our future and if we don't help them now, the consequences will be felt for generations to come.***

Growing Up Healthy will show you how nutrients work to prevent disease and how diseases may progress without the benefit of healthy lifestyle habits. It will also show you how to help your children develop a healthy lifestyle. The book includes:

- a step-by-step behavioral plan to guide you in making a habit of eating healthy foods and exercising regularly,

- an innovative, easy-to-follow nutrition plan suitable for everyone, and

- a DVD that teaches children resistance training exercises and aerobic exercises.

Although the Next Generation Fitness Program is designed for children, a healthy lifestyle is important for everyone— children, adolescents, parents and even grandparents. Everyone can benefit from healthier eating habits and regular exercise. The nutrition program is unique in its ability to satisfy your nutritional needs and your palate, keep you at a healthy weight and provide you with more energy. The exercise program will increase your metabolic rate, improve muscle mass, help increase bone mass and improve your overall feeling of well-being. Next Generation Fitness is a program that can and should be followed for life!

chapter one

The Unhealthy Child— A New Epidemic

People around the world are exposed to more and more nutritionally deficient foods, creating an increasingly unhealthy population.[1] We are exposed to hundreds of thousands of processed foods. Every day our children are bombarded with ads for very unhealthy foods; then they are served these foods in school, at parties, at the homes of friends, in restaurants and even in our own homes. These foods have caused an alarming increase in overweight, obesity and poor eating habits.

The obesity epidemic is frightening, especially when we look at the statistics for children. Sixteen percent of children between the ages of 6-19 are overweight, a number that has more than tripled since 1980.[2] (SEE APPENDIX 1.) The medical community does not have an answer to this problem. But an obvious solution is to get our children off the computers and videogames and outdoors, and to teach them about healthy food choices. Some organizations and school systems are trying to address this issue and have taken the initiative by promoting physical education programs and after-school sports. There is also a trend toward establishing guidelines for offering more nutritious foods in school cafeterias. However, the process of making systemic changes that can contribute to the solution of this problem is very slow. The real key to solving the problem lies in the family. Together, parents and children need to learn how to deal with the plethora of non-nutritious foods advertised at every turn and prominently displayed in stores as well as the constant lure of videogames and computers. Parents are the role models for their children; if parents adopt a healthy lifestyle, their children will naturally follow it.

Proper nutrition and a healthier lifestyle must start at a young age. If we help children develop good habits when they are young, the possibility of decreasing future morbidity and mortality is astounding.[3] The younger children are when they develop good habits, the more likely it is that these habits will stay with them throughout life.

Staying healthy requires goal setting, meal planning, understanding the benefits of good foods and exercise and integrating this knowledge into everyday behavior. Children cannot do this alone; they need family participation. Parents must participate with their children in this program to increase the chances of children becoming healthy adults. It is never too late to start or too early to begin; babies, children, adolescents and adults can all benefit from the healthy habits described in this program. If followed correctly, the Next Generation Fitness Program will lead to a much healthier life, one with more energy and vigor, a greater ability to learn and less risk of disease.

Research has shown that certain food nutrients have a protective effect in preventing heart disease, type II diabetes, infections, inflammation, stroke, high blood pressure, cancers and dementia.[4] Plant-derived nutrients, also known as phytonutrients, are found in abundance in fruits, vegetables, legumes, nuts and whole grains. However, some of these nutrients are lost when food is processed. Even though over 8,000 food nutrients have been identified, we are depriving our bodies of them because so many of the foods we eat are processed.[5] The easy availability of processed, high-fat, quick foods results in our children growing up without the benefit of the protection offered by these nutrients. This has created a generation of unhealthy children.

Children are more likely to have low blood levels of micronutrients—the minerals that our body needs, like selenium, chromium, zinc, etc.—as well as phytonutrients because children are filling themselves with non-nutrient-dense foods. These low blood levels are not life threatening, as a vitamin C deficiency might be, but they can be life altering nonetheless. Without these protective phytonutrients and micronutrients our bodies are more at risk for many diseases. A call to action has been taken by the Center for Disease Control as well as the World Health Organization, to name a few of the public health agencies that are sounding alarms.[6] This call to action involves getting our children to eat more fruits and vegetables and to get more exercise. It has been estimated that altering one's diet and exercising regularly have the potential to decrease the rate of heart disease by 80 percent, type II diabetes by 90 percent and cancer by 30 percent![7] All we need to do is get our children exercising and eating more fruits and vegetables.

Defining Health

In order to fully understand the ramifications of this epidemic and just how unhealthy it is, it is important to know what is considered healthy. The dictionary definition of health is to be "sound in body" or "free from disease." Since these definitions are somewhat vague, let me explain what I consider to be a healthy child. A healthy child is one who is free from disease; has an appropriate intake of calories in the form of fruits, vegetables, legumes, lean meats and whole grains; AND expends a proper amount of energy in the form of cardiac-stimulating activity and resistance training.

As a pediatrician, I deal with children's illness as well as their health. To evaluate a child's health, of course, I examine the child. But I also always ask both the parent and the child a lot of questions to help me assess the three most important variables: the child's height and weight, the child's nutritional intake and the child's physical activity. The basic questions involve what the child is eating and what kind and how much exercise the child is getting. Although the answers I get to these questions can be both funny and sad, they also give me a window into the child's overall health-related habits. Lifestyle habits can't be solved by one talk with a child's doctor, but it is a good place to start. Assuming that a child is free from obvious disease, 80 percent of my time during a check-up is spent evaluating these three factors.

HEIGHT/WEIGHT

The first thing I look at during a check-up is the child's height and weight. These simple numeric values are very important in revealing the overall picture of the health of the child. These numbers can tell me whether a child has gained too much or too little weight in relationship to the increase in height. If a child gains too little weight and has not grown much in height, it usually is a sign that something more serious is going on and steps need to be taken to find the cause of the problem. Alternatively, if a child has gained too much weight, this also needs to be evaluated. All too frequently, this is the problem.

The weight and height parameters are used together to calculate the body mass index or BMI. The BMI is a ratio of weight to height and it is being used more and more frequently as a standard way to measure a healthy body weight. An adult BMI should fall between 19 kg/m^2 and 25 kg/m^2. A BMI over 25 is defined as overweight; greater than 30 is, by definition, considered obese. A child's BMI alone cannot determine whether or not the child is overweight. Therefore, for children doctors also use standardized charts that plot BMI and age and give the results as a percentile range. The normal range is from 5-85 percent. If a child's BMI plots between the 85th percentile and the 95th percentile, the child is considered at risk for becoming overweight. Oftentimes, parents may be completely unaware that their child is at risk for becoming overweight. Once a child is above the 95th percentile, the child is officially overweight. Whether the child is at risk for overweight or officially overweight, the issue needs to be addressed during the child's check-up. But we need to **avoid** getting to this point. I can never overemphasize that eating healthy foods and exercising regularly will ensure a healthier future for your child.[8]

When monitoring a child's growth and health, it is important to watch for percentile changes in the child's BMI. If a child has been at the 20th percentile for years and suddenly jumps to the 75th percentile, bells should go off. It is time to take a serious look at the child's food intake and exercise output. The same applies to the child who has had a normal BMI that suddenly falls into a much lower percentile. Although the growth percentiles for a child change, and this is a normal part of growth, when such change becomes a steady trend, it needs to be evaluated.

There are some caveats when evaluating a child's BMI. There are children who have a significant amount of muscle mass and therefore have an elevated BMI. This occurs in very muscular boys and girls as well as in body builders. These children would certainly not be considered overweight, so we need to look at another parameter—their waist circumference. A large waist circumference, along with an elevated BMI, means that the child is in the overweight category. Again there are no single numbers to define an enlarged waist circumference for children, as there are for adults (adult males should have a waist circumference less than 40 inches; females should be less than 35 inches), but there are standardized graphs that show the normal ranges for different ages. Most pediatricians are able to identify children who are overweight without the use of charts. An enlarged waist circumference is associated with an increased risk of heart disease and should set off alarms; immediate action should be taken to begin a healthier lifestyle. This applies to adults as well as children.

It is important to mention another related issue: We live in a society that places too much emphasis on what a person looks like and not enough emphasis on being **healthy**. Many parents who bring in their children for wellness check-ups are very worried about how their child looks. They may have noticed that their child is getting bigger; they also may have noted an increase in fat distribution throughout the child's body. Many children start to change shape just before the onset of puberty and parents naturally are concerned when any unexpected change occurs in their child. It is important to remember that a wide range of body weights are considered normal. People who eat right and exercise daily come in all different shapes and sizes. They may not fit the Hollywood definition of body beautiful, but they are certainly healthy, and that is what really counts. If my patient is eating healthy foods, taking in an adequate amount of calories, avoiding junk foods and exercising regularly, I will reassure the parent that these healthy habits will stick with the child; most likely the child will not have a problem with weight. However, follow-up is needed at regular intervals so I can continue to monitor the child.

On the other side of the spectrum, we should not presume that because some people are naturally thin, they are healthy. If your child is thin, or you as a parent are thin, your body still needs the right foods and daily physical activity to maintain good health. Filling a thin body with junk food and avoiding exercise because your weight is stable, still leaves you with an increased risk for disease. Even people who do not have a weight problem should follow a healthy nutrition plan and exercise routine, allowing for additional **healthy** food servings to maintain a proper weight. What a person looks like is not nearly as important as lifestyle habits.

NUTRITIONAL INTAKE

A simple question that I ask children at each check up is, "Are you eating your fruits and vegetables everyday?" Most children will respond with a vigorous affirmative nod while the parent stands behind the child nodding no. I will then ask the child exactly what fruits and vegetables he or she is eating. At this point, many children will make a face and tell me that they don't like vegetables or say they "ate an apple last week." Most children will go on to tell me of the foods that they "tried" in the vegetable category; some will even tell me of the fruits they eat regularly. It is the rare patient who reports eating fruits AND vegetables everyday. It's not surprising that some parents are frustrated with trying to get their children to eat better. I have even had parents ask me if any child really eats what they're supposed to each day. Well, there are some children who eat the recommended daily servings of fruits and vegetables—about 20 percent in the U.S. We need to get that number closer to 100 percent!

Pediatricians have special relationships with their patients. We care for children from infancy to early adulthood and sometimes we are the only doctor they know. This can put pediatricians in a very powerful position. If we have done a good job and have built a trusting relationship, children will listen to what we tell them. In addition, since we are dealing with children, parents often seek advice about their child. I am always happy to give it. However, time is limited during doctor visits and so many things need to be accomplished. I therefore make a point of telling every parent, child and adolescent to make sure they are eating fruits and vegetables EVERY DAY. Children often will take my advice and very proudly report back to me on their newly acquired dietary habits. This is a great feeling of accomplishment for me because I know what a dramatic impact these food changes will have on their future.

Children are amazing learners and are always eager to listen. During the talks in my office with patients and their families, I also discuss how much food is an appropriate amount to eat each day. (Food quantities and portions are discussed in more detail in Chapter Six.) This often reinforces what most parents are trying to do at home. For those parents who have not been thinking about dietary habits, these talks help them become aware of the relationship between what we eat and their child's future health and the importance of food choices in our daily lives.

PHYSICAL ACTIVITY

The benefits of daily exercise are well-documented.[9] The reduction in heart disease, some cancers and hypertension are just a few of the diseases that we know can be prevented through regular exercise.[10] Other benefits include improved bone density, a stronger immune system, sounder sleep, increased energy, improved coordination, increased self-esteem and improved ability to concentrate in school.[11] In addition, daily exercise can help reduce the incidence of obesity.[12]

When I ask my patients about exercise, the most common response often consists of a description of how the child plays on a sports team, whether soccer, baseball, football, lacrosse or other sports. The majority of teams meet twice a week, once for practice and once for the game. Not only is this too little exercise, but sports teams are not designed to get the child into the HABIT of exercise. Team sports concentrate on sport-specific skills, not lifelong exercise habits. There are children who are very involved in highly competitive sports teams and these children usually get plenty of exercise during the week. However, we still need to make sure that exercise becomes a habitual part of children's lives so that once the sport season is over, exercising does not come to a complete halt.

We can do this by teaching children how to exercise at ***home***. Most parents don't realize that their children should be exercising at home, regardless of the extent of their sports activities. Furthermore, they are not aware that children also should be doing resistance training for maximal benefit.

Sports team activities rarely teach children about resistance training. The importance of resistance training has been over-looked because it was once thought that this type of training might be harmful for growing children. In the past, some doctors where worried that weight training could harm the growing skeleton and possibly "stunt growth." Using any type of exercise equipment inappropriately will increase anybody's chance for injury—not just children. The Next Generation Fitness exercise program uses the only natural way to resistance train: using the child's body weight as the resistance. There is no better way to build muscle and improve bone strength than to use a child's body weight as the resistant force; there is no worry about a weight being too heavy and damaging a finger or worse yet loosing a finger to the weight stack. Unfortunately, children are accidents waiting to happen when they are unsupervised in gyms. I do not recommend children using weight rooms. Resistance training is a crucial part of any exercise program and we are now aware of all the benefits to the growing muscles and skeleton.[13] Resistance training should be an integral part of our exercise routine for maximal benefit.

Home exercise is essential, first because exercising should be convenient and readily accessible. You do not need fancy equip-ment or a gym to get a great workout. It is sometimes not feasi-ble for people to go out to a gym and it creates a reason to avoid exercising altogether. It is also very important for children to get in the habit of exercising. As children go through high school, there is a natural attrition rate in their participation in organized sports. The situation gets even worse when they go to college. If children are not taught how to exercise without a team, they are not likely to continue to exercise. On the other hand, if parents instill the *habit* of exercise at home, without fancy equipment, children will automatically continue to exercise long after they have discontinued participating in team sports.

chapter two

The Road to the Solution

Obesity and excess weight is a serious problem in both adults and children not only in the U.S. but in many other parts of the world. More and more people are dying from preventable diseases like coronary heart disease, diabetes, stroke and cancers. Most Americans are overweight and children are getting heavier every year.[1]

The first step to solving this health crisis is identifying and understanding the causes. But this is only one piece of the puzzle. Although the problem has been identified and most of us know how to avoid these ills, we are not using the knowledge we have to turn this trend around. Taking the action needed to successfully conquer the problem will take effort. If parents are able to change their lifestyle for the better, they can be assured that their efforts will be well spent: their children will have a healthier future.[2]

We are surrounded by messages that stress the importance of eating good foods and staying fit. So why don't most people do it? There are several reasons. We are also inundated with messages that tempt us with junk foods, and fast foods are often very convenient. In addition, the consequences of not eating right and staying fit are not usually immediate; since they are long-term, we tend not to pay attention to them on a day-to-day basis. But an even bigger reason is that most people are not really aware of why it is so important to eat good foods and stay fit. Of course we know that it is healthier, but knowing something on an intellectual level is not the same thing as actually having an internal understanding that we act on. Let me try to explain the difference. We know that too much sun can be dangerous so most people use sunscreen when they spend time in the sun. We associate sunburn and excess exposure to the sun with skin cancer and we are usually careful about protecting ourselves. Because we understand and believe in the causal relationship, we act on it, and we protect our children with sunscreen as well. A similar understanding is needed with diet, nutrition and exercise.

Being aware of why eating well is so important involves understanding how food nutrients work inside our bodies. Let me start by addressing how food nutrients affect our health. It would be impossible to describe the more than 8,000 phytonutrients found in the foods we eat, but it is important to understand some of the major ones and the effects they have on our bodies.

We hear so much about ***antioxidants*** and how important it is to get them in our diet, but many people have no idea of what they are and how they work. In order to understand antioxidants, we first need to understand the term free radical. Free radicals are highly charged and unstable molecules that are produced naturally in the cells of our body as a result of daily metabolic functioning. Charged molecules naturally seek stability by taking electrons from any available source. The most readily available sources in the body are found in the cellular membranes and DNA. Here's an analogy that I often use to help explain this concept to my patients and their families. Think of your body as a pinball machine and the free radicals as the pinballs. Just like a pinball that bounces frenetically inside the pinball machine, free radicals bounce around in the bloodstream causing damage to blood vessels, cell membranes and DNA. When DNA is damaged, it can set off a series of events that could lead to cancer.

Antioxidants are substances that inhibit the reactions of free radicals. Our bodies need a constant supply of antioxidants to counter the effects of the free radicals and keep us healthy. The more antioxidants in the blood, the less likely it is that free radicals will build up and cause damage and disease. An altered balance between free radicals and the antioxidants that squelch them causes what's known as oxidative stress: there are more free radicals than the body can handle. This situation can increase the risk of acquiring many diseases.[3]

Production of free radicals is increased by a diet high in saturated fat, smoking, stress, pollution, radiation, inflammation, infection and even intense exercise. Free radicals are also generated from the normal, everyday cellular reactions that keep the body functioning. Eating foods that contain antioxidants ensures that the free radicals are neutralized as our body produces them, thereby decreasing the risk of disease. Most phytonutrients have antioxidant properties, which is one of the reasons that these plant-derived nutrients have so much power in preventing disease. The phytonutrients found in fruits, vegetables, legumes, whole grains and teas contain high levels of antioxidants.

Understanding the role that free radicals play in causing disease and the power that antioxidants provide in clearing these molecules from the body is the first step in improving your family's diet. The next step is to really internalize this knowledge so that living a healthy lifestyle is as automatic and natural as applying sunscreen before a day at the beach.

First form a mental picture of free radicals bouncing around inside your body causing damage. Then picture antioxidants snuffing them out, like Pac-Man gobbling up the little dots. Do this mental exercise whenever you are eating. If you are eating a nutrient-filled meal, picture the destruction of the free radicals; if you are eating a nutrient-deficient meal (like a burger and fries), picture the free radicals bouncing around and causing damage to cells and DNA. Eating meals high in fat and sugar throws the

body into oxidative stress because of the excess free radicals produced by such foods. Many children walk around in a state of
oxidative stress because of poor nutrition. On a day-to-day basis
you may not notice any change externally in your child. When
the body has been in an oxidative stress state for extended
periods of time, however, the condition may be more apparent;
your child may be more susceptible to picking up illnesses, have
more difficulty concentrating, have less energy than normal or
be more irritable. Think about the damage this is causing!
Visualizing what happens inside your body on a regular basis
will help you not only understand the power of nutrition but
also help you to take protective action.

There are also classes of phytonutrients that have been
shown to inhibit cancer cell growth, destroy cancer cells, activate
our own cancer defense system or deactivate cancer causing
agents (mutagens). Some examples of cancer-fighting foods
include broccoli and onions. Broccoli contains a phytonutrient
called sulforaphane, which has been shown to destroy some
cancer cells in the laboratory.[4] Onions contain organosulfur
compounds, which also have been shown to inhibit cancer
cell growth.[5]

Another phytonutrient that has received much attention is
lycopene. Lycopene has multiple, inherent anticancer properties;
it inhibits cancer cell growth and prevents normal cells from
turning into cancer cells. Lycopene is a very powerful antioxidant
that tends to concentrate itself in the body, and in particular, in
prostate tissue. In fact, lycopene has been shown to decrease the
incidence of prostate cancer.[6] If you eat foods that contain
lycopene on a regular basis, free radicals that are formed in the
prostate gland are neutralized quickly by the antioxidants and
thus are not around to cause damage to DNA and potentially set
off a tumor gene. As a matter of fact lycopene is so effective in
helping to prevent prostate cancer that studies are underway
using lycopene as an adjuvant to therapy for prostate cancer![7]

Tomatoes contain a particularly high level of lycopene, but it is also found in pink grapefruit, watermelon, papaya and apricots. Lycopene is what gives the red color to these foods.

Other phytonutrients have the power to prevent the growth of cancer cells before they even become a problem by cutting off the blood supply to the cancer cells. There are many more advantages to phytonutrients that are just being discovered: some have anti-inflammatory properties, some can inhibit bacterial growth, stimulate the immune system and decrease platelet stickiness.[8] Decreasing platelet stickiness decreases clogging of the arteries and helps to keep blood vessels smooth, reducing the danger of a heart attack or stroke.

While reading about the power of food nutrients and how they work is an important first step, in order to make the lifestyle changes necessary to act on this information, we have to really internalize that understanding and adopt a healthy lifestyle. In my experience, using visualization techniques puts you on your way to processing the knowledge and owning it. If we visualize food nutrients on a molecular level, we can create an image of the molecules at work destroying potential cancer cells or activating the body's cancer defense system. This kind of thinking goes a long way toward helping us process our knowledge of nutrition.

Try this mental exercise: Visualize your blood flowing tumultuously through vessels that have bumps filled with plaque (thick patches of fatty deposits inside blood vessels). The blood cannot flow smoothly because of the plaque, causing some turbulence in blood flow. When this happens, the sticky platelets start to form clots inside the blood vessels. This series of events can lead to heart attack, stroke, dementia and acute death. Now visualize your blood flowing through the same blood vessels also filled with areas of plaque. But because you are eating a diet filled with phytonutrients, your platelets are less sticky and clots do not form. The blood flows through the vessels bringing oxygen to its destination!

Let's take this visualization to another level. Instead of your own body, picture what is going on inside your child's body when he or she is eating deep fried chicken nuggets with French fries. Remember the LACK of antioxidants in these foods and then think about your child's body filling up with free radicals bouncing around and causing cell damage because the meal was devoid of any real nutrition; in fact, the meal was filled with saturated fat that ***increased*** the body's free radical content. Once you have created such a frightening image of your child's body, it is easier to be motivated to make sure your children get phytonutrients on a daily basis. We would never intentionally do harm to our children, so why would we let them fill their bodies with foods that research has shown to be bad for them? It just takes understanding of how phytonutrients work and owning that knowledge so we act on it automatically.

I know that using visualization techniques work. Of course I do not want parents to create frightening mental images of their children, but I do want parents to truly understand how food can alter their child's life and live by that recognition. Healthy food will change things for the better, but a poor diet will cause damage and is likely to lead to medical problems as the child grows. If you truly believe this, it will be much easier to transition your family to learning how to eat and exercise for life.

It is important to review this information to keep knowledge about the power of phytonutrients in the foreground. Try to do the visualization exercises as much as you can. Become conscious of what is going on inside your body when you eat certain foods. Once this starts to become a habit, you will begin to find yourself in the believing stage, where you have internalized the information. When we believe something, we ***accept it as true or real.*** If knowledge is not turned into true belief, it is merely an intellectual exercise. We need to believe things on a conscious and subconscious level to achieve automatic action. It is very important to truly believe that improving your family's lifestyle habits will affect their future health. Without this belief, trying to change your child's habits will be much less effective; children can always sense when parents give mixed signals, which is common when they are not committed to something. All parents have been victims of their own lack of conviction when it comes to dealing with their children (how many times have you given in to buying a toy because your child nagged you?). Children are often very intuitive about their parents; they sense when their parents are weak and will give in and when they won't budge because there is no ambivalence. Parents cannot afford to be weak when it comes to their children's lifestyle health habits because their future depends on it.

It seems apparent that although many adults know that eating a high-fat diet and avoiding exercise will cause them tremendous pain in the future, they have not internalized the connection. Roughly 25 percent of adults consume the recommended number of servings of fruits and vegetables each day.[9] At the same time we are consuming so much processed, fatty food that the vast majority of the population is quickly becoming overweight. Eating needs to be a pleasurable experience but it never has to be an unhealthy experience. Unfortunately for many people, it has become just that. This needs to change if we want to lead productive, long lives.

You must believe in something to make changes and you must connect the habit to its consequences in the present and the future. For example, there are people who know that smoking is dangerous but they continue to smoke. These same people would not jump out of a moving train or otherwise risk their lives for a frivolous cause, yet they will continue to puff on those cigarettes. Why? Because they don't really think that what they are doing will result in lung cancer or cause them to have a heart attack. They don't connect the consequences of their present behavior to their own future health. If smokers were to visualize the one billion free radicals formed with ***each puff*** on their cigarette, or chest pain that requires a trip to the hospital or dying before ever getting to know their grandchildren, it might have an impact. Get smokers to think of these things every day and it certainly will have an effect on them; when these concepts become a part of their conscious and subconscious thinking, they will **believe that smoking could kill them**. Once smokers believe this, they will be able to make a change and quit.

Internalizing and believing are such important concepts in our lives because they allow us to make changes. Every parent needs to believe in the benefits of nutrition and exercise. Telling your child to eat fruits and vegetables every day is not enough to get them to eat them. We try to teach our children to eat well because we know it is the correct thing to do, but if we really don't believe that there is a significant benefit in eating fruits and vegetables or if we don't believe that there is great danger in consuming junk foods regularly, how can we expect our children to follow our advice? As a parent, however, if you truly believe that eating well can prevent disease, you will be better equipped to ensure that you and your family get the proper nutrition.

In my pediatric practice, parents often talk to me about their child's eating habits. They will tell me that they can't get their child to eat vegetables, or the child will only eat two or three different foods. (Note: For children who are developmentally delayed, autistic or psychologically troubled, trying to ensure that they eat well may cause too much added stress to an already difficult situation; in these cases, nutrition will temporarily take a backseat until the other more life-altering issues have been handled.) Often parents are hoping to find a quick solution to the problem. However, I can't give them a solution until they really believe that they have a problem. Most parents know that it is better to have a balanced diet, but they will still give their child the same three foods over and over again simply because the child wants them; they will insist that the child won't eat anything else. These parents do not truly believe that this behavior will have life-altering effects on their children. We know that parents would never let their child go to school without a coat on a freezing day because the parents **believe** that this behavior could result in harm to their child. In this situation, the parents don't just intellectually understand the importance of weather-appropriate clothing for the child, the parents truly believe that wearing a coat on a freezing day is mandatory; there is no discussion about it. Similarly, parents would certainly rectify the situation if they thought their child would be harmed by perpetually poor eating. If we are secure in our knowledge of something, we will act on it.

Now we need to apply the same principles to exercise. Why do so many people avoid physical activity? The benefits of exercise go way beyond keeping your heart healthy; some of them can be immediately felt and quickly noticed.[10] Most people experience a feeling of well being after a good workout. They get an exercise "high." This is because exercise stimulates the release of endorphins, the body's natural feel-good hormones. In addition, most people notice an improvement in their physical appearance soon after they begin regular exercise. They sleep better, look better, have more energy and at the same time, they are increasing their life span. Alluring as these things are, for most people they are not enough to get them into the habit of exercise. The main excuses I hear people use to avoid exercise is they do not have the time, they are too tired, they can't get started or it is not fun. Identifying the reasons can lead to a solution.

Among all the excuses, lack of the motivation to start to exercise is the biggest obstacle. Motivation naturally follows once you really believe that exercise will add life to your years as well as years to your life. To help get over the motivation hurdle, visualize a more energetic, leaner and stronger you. Then visualize a long life that does not slow to a stop, but keeps going with a sharp mind and body. Think about being able to teach your grandchildren to ski, hike and ride a bike. Motivation can also come from visualizing what the future will be like without the benefit of regular exercise in your life. Create a mental picture of yourself getting older and succumbing to heart disease, or stroke, or cancer or dementia. Picture this happening to your children as they grow older. The last thing parents want is to see their child become debilitated by poor health. While exercise cannot guarantee that you'll never be affected by disease, it does have a protective effect and it does lower the risk. A lifetime without exercise will cause your life to slow down rapidly because of poor stamina, osteoporosis, decreased muscle mass and brain deterioration.[11] The mental exercise of seeing your future with and without physical exercise is highly motivational for most people. But remember, *all visualizations need to be practiced regularly* so that they become internalized.

Making time for exercise needs to be a priority, but it does not need to interrupt your day. The thought of taking a 30-45 minute chunk out of your day may seem impossible, but exercising does not need to be done all at once. Solving the time problem is easier if you break up exercise into small, bite-size pieces. Exercising in front of the television is not unreasonable. Most families find time to watch television together. Take some of this time to sit on the floor and do some exercises. Taking 10-15 minutes to do some sit ups, push ups and jumping jacks in the morning and evening is a great way for both children and adults to start and end their day. For adults, take another 15-30 minutes to take a brisk walk during your lunch hour. Make sure children get plenty of outside running and playing every day. All of us have small bits of time to devote to exercise. We just need to make it a priority.

Enjoying a workout is not always so easy. Many people have good exercise habits but do not enjoy working out. They are disciplined and they focus on the results—the exercise "high" and how good they are going to feel after their workout. They remind themselves that this is the "price they have to pay to keep fit." But this does NOT have to be the case. Exercising can be fun and should involve the whole family. Planning regular activities like biking, swimming, hiking or walking is a fun way to keep fit. If scheduling enough time for such activities is a problem, create routines that use smaller chunks of time. Get your children to start a morning and evening exercise routine, but make it fun! You must vibrate enthusiasm and fun when exercising with your children. Using a visualization technique at this point may help generate enthusiasm. Picture yourself as a leaner, more energetic, playful and productive person; imagine yourself laughing with your children as you exercise. Enthusiasm is catching and children can sense when a parent is having fun working out; they too will soon enjoy it. As your children grow up, they will associate exercise with happy times with their family, and their subsequent workouts will always be fun!

Many people tell me they are "too tired to work out," but part of the reason that they are tired is because they are not physically fit. This is a vicious cycle: You don't exercise because you are too tired, but you will be tired if you don't start to exercise. Start working out in small, bite-size pieces, and your energy level will naturally improve, making exercising easier. As you get into shape, regular exercise becomes a habit that you can't avoid—you start to crave it and feel unsatisfied if you miss a few days. The exercise *habit* needs to be instilled in all children; once it does we can achieve our goals: a healthier life for ourselves and our families.

Here are some facts that can help support and motivate you to begin a healthier lifestyle:

- The chance of our children getting some cancers can be reduced by 30 percent if they eat the recommended amount of vegetables each day.[12]

- Our children will increase their lifespan if they eat more fruits and vegetables.[13]

- Children will have an increased risk of heart disease before the age of 50 if they never learn how to exercise routinely.[14]

- The chances of our children getting osteoporosis as adults can be reduced by making sure they get enough calcium AND by doing resistance exercises.[15]

- Altering our lifestyle could prevent 64 percent of the diseases in the world.[16]

- Five out of six chronic diseases can be prevented by practicing good health habits.[17]

- If we don't make changes in our daily health habits, 90 percent of the population will soon be overweight.[18]

Use these facts to create personalized visualizations about food nutrients, exercise and good health habits. It is only when we start to really believe that these facts directly affect us that we can begin to change our habits. This is important not only for ourselves but for the future of our children.

chapter three

The Steps to a Healthy Generation

The best preventative medicine of the 21st century is proper nutrition and exercise. Now that you know why it is so important to eat well and exercise regularly, you need to set your mind to changing those habits that are harming rather than helping you and your family. I know that raising children who have great health habits is not always so easy. The hardest part is getting children to break their old habits and form new, healthy ones.

I have spent my life developing healthy habits for myself and my children. Since I did not grow up with the best nutrition and exercise habits, I first had to teach them to myself. My children, however, have the advantage of growing up with these healthy habits so they will not have to make any major adjustments as they grow older. What a great gift to give to your children! Because eating nutritious foods and exercising on a regular basis have become habits, they require no effort or thought. These things can and should become as much a part of our everyday routines as brushing our teeth. The younger children are when they are surrounded by good habits, the easier it is for them to acquire them. The goal is for these habits to continue through succeeding generations.

Taking the steps to secure a healthy future for your child requires thoughtful planning and a core belief that you are doing the absolute best for your child. Breaking old habits can be difficult and busy families understandably have trouble finding extra time. Parents look for foods that are quick and easy to prepare and are often additionally hampered by the limited foods that their children will eat. But giving in to fast food restaurants, which offer convenient, tasty, high-fat foods, creates a problem. Children quickly acquire a taste for these high-fat foods, and then they are not usually even willing to try foods that look different and especially taste different. We need to make changes! Remember that if you are not committed to making sure your child gets the proper nutrition and exercise each day, you will not be successful. The following steps work very well in ensuring success, but each one must be followed. As you look at each step, start to plan how you will change your family's future.

Anticipate

The first step toward healthier eating is to ANTICIPATE the effects of unhealthy eating and lack of exercise and act early to foster healthy habits. As we have seen, the consequences of not acting on our knowledge about health can be profound. Knowing this, the time to start is now, regardless of how old your children are and what kind of habits your family has. Like adults, children are creatures of habit. We take delight in how quickly they absorb everything around them. They imitate our expressions, language and actions and quickly pick up our habits, both good and bad. Breaking habits is not easy for anyone, so we need to ANTICIPATE the reactions of our children and be prepared if they balk at the change. This is a challenge for every parent, especially if you are also trying to change your own habits at the same time. I have counseled parents who battle with their children over food and eating habits, though it should not be a battle. At times it is much easier to give in and say yes but herein lays the food challenge.

Parents love to see the joy on their child's face as he or she opens a present or eats a favorite ice cream. Of course we get pleasure out of making our children happy and we never want them to feel bad. So we often give in to them to avoid the tears that follow a "no." As parents, we have to put limitations on everything; when few limits are set, a problem usually arises. When parents fail to set limits early in their child's development, they leave themselves vulnerable to even larger problems later on. Parents need to be aware of the long-term results as well as the short-term gains. We need to ANTICIPATE the consequences of not setting limits and saying no. Being prepared to foster healthy habits while children are young is the first step to a healthier adulthood.

Parents may not be aware that feeding their child junk food is actually harmful to them. We already know that we need to both understand and believe that poor lifestyle habits have ramifications that go far beyond childhood years. Parents know that eating fruits and vegetables is good for their children and they often think that it would be better of course if their children ate healthier foods. What they often do not realize, however, is that **not** eating fruits and vegetables may actually be harming their children. Let me give you an example. I have a patient who is afflicted with renal tubular acidosis and requires medication four times a day to prevent progression of the disease. If her medication is **not** given to her for a day or two, or some doses are skipped occasionally, there are no noticeable changes. However, if her medication were to be skipped frequently, she would slowly experience growth problems and bony rickets, conditions that would be with her for life. This is the same disease that afflicted Tiny Tim in Charles Dickens' *A Christmas Carol*. Luckily, today we have medication that can prevent this disease from progressing. I don't know of any parent of such a child who would think that this medication was optional. Think of healthy foods as good medicine; they can prevent many diseases. Chronic ingestion of unhealthy foods and lack of exercise will not necessarily be evident immediately, but they are still harmful. Eating junk food and ***not*** eating fruits and vegetables are both detrimental to your health.

Ideally, we should ANTICIPATE the consequences of eating unhealthy foods when our children are very young. Babies start to eat table food around the age of 9 months and parents can begin to introduce healthy new foods and tastes. Babies often play with their food and may even throw it on the floor. This is not a sign that the baby does not like the food; the baby is merely enjoying experimenting with what happens when objects are dropped. Parents are still very much in control of their child's food intake at this point, and it is the best stage at which to start healthy eating patterns.

Starting table foods (finger foods) is a crucial time in a baby's life. ***Only*** healthy foods should be introduced to the developing child. These foods will include fresh soft fruits; well-cooked vegetables; soft, whole grain foods; legumes and lean meats. If a baby only knows the tastes of healthy foods, he or she becomes accustomed to them early on, and these will remain the child's taste preferences even in adulthood.

It's useful to remember that children's tastes change and such changes can seem sudden. This is normal. If your child loved broccoli but suddenly refuses to eat it, do not offer an unhealthy food just to get the child to eat. Because parents are terrified at the thought of their child not eating, they sometimes feel compelled to offer unhealthy alternatives because they know the child will eat them, for example processed food or junk food. Unfortunately, this is a common mistake and doing this is worse than having a child go to bed hungry. If your child decides he or she does not like broccoli anymore, then offer a healthy substitute (for example, cauliflower), but still keep broccoli on the menu. If the child continues to refuse to eat broccoli, there are many healthy alternatives. The food choices that we give babies and toddlers have a tremendous impact on their future health. We must always keep this in mind if we start to feel guilty. By not giving in to providing junk food as an option (chicken nuggets, hot dogs, etc.), you have anticipated the effects of these foods and you have done what is best for your child.

Some parents worry that being firm about food choices will create an eating disorder. This is not the case. You are not going to battle with your child—you are just giving your child healthy choices. You can't (and shouldn't try to) force a child to eat! If you start to demand that your child clean the plate or eat *one* particular food, *you will always lose*. As the parent, you give the choices and the child decides which of those choices to eat. This gives some control to the child while maintaining limits.

From the very beginning, it is crucial that you set the rules. It is easy to offer only healthy food choices to a baby; this will be the only thing the baby knows and he or she will be completely content. However, as children get older and are exposed to the junk food world, our job gets a bit harder. When children are in school or at a friend's home, we have no control over the foods they are offered and what they choose to eat. Nevertheless, if parents follow all of the steps in the Next Generation Fitness Program, their child will be armed with good eating habits and will be more likely to make healthier choices in these situations.

Let me give you an example of how failure to ANTICIPATE can cause a major eating problem. I was performing a check-up on an 18-month-old and inquired about the child's eating. The mother told me that her son would only eat fast-food chicken nuggets (and only from one particular fast-food restaurant, at that!) for dinner. She was tired of going out every night to buy the chicken nuggets but was terrified that if she didn't, her son would not get enough protein. So she gave in to the child's demands and her child ate high-fat, non-nutrient filled chicken nuggets every night for dinner. I informed the mother that her behavior was doing more harm than good and reassured her that her son would never starve himself; all she needed to do was offer healthier dinner choices and not give in to his demands. She immediately took my advice and stopped giving him the chicken nuggets. There were a few days when the child did not eat dinner and cried in protest, but eventually he started to eat what his mother offered for dinner. Because this parent started giving in to the child's wishes, dinnertime had turned into a big chore, creating a situation in which the child made the rules and the parent acceded to the child's demands. An 18-month-old surely is not old enough to decide what to eat for dinner every night. This mother failed to ANTICIPATE what would happen if she introduced unhealthy foods to her child at such an early age. The child developed a taste for the unhealthy food at a time when his taste preferences were developing and he lost interest in other foods. Because the mother continued to give in, she lost control of the situation.

If your children are older and refuse to eat any vegetables and/or fruits, we have some work to do. It is likely that you will meet some resistance if you suddenly give your child only healthy choices. It is important to know that children will start to acquire a taste for any food when they are continually exposed to it over a short period of time. Research has shown that it takes children a minimum of ten food exposures over a two-week period before they acquire a taste for a new food.[1] So be patient and persistent. For example, to introduce spinach into the diet, be prepared to insist that your child taste it each night you offer it. The child does not have to eat it if he or she doesn't like it, but make it a rule that the child has to at least *taste* it. Making sure that children take a taste of a particular food is much different from forcing them to eat it or clean their plates, and it is important to understand the difference. The child has the choice of whether or not to eat the food after tasting it; it is the child who has the final decision. If you offer your child a spinach dish prepared differently every night for two weeks and insist that the child taste it, after the two weeks, *your child will willingly eat the spinach!* There are certain things that we must make sure our children do. For example, they must do their homework or at least try to do it. If they need help, a parent is always available. The same holds true for new foods; children may not arbitrarily refuse to eat a new food. They must try them, but they do not have to eat them. This policy ensures that there are no battles about food and that children are exposed to all kinds of healthy food options.

Time for family eating is very important. Another part of anticipation involves thinking about family meals ahead of time. This will be time well spent since it can ensure that you have only healthy choices available at home. It also helps to keep nutrition on your mind so you can shop accordingly. Sometimes it helps to prepare lunches and dinners ahead of time so that you're not tempted to resort to fast food alternatives. You may even want to review the school lunch menu with your children and help them choose only the healthy foods. If there are none, talk to the school and try to make some changes.

There are many families today who because of parent work schedules do not have the time to prepare meals, so they frequently go out to eat. Remember, most restaurants always have at least a few healthy items on the menu. Look over the menus carefully, point out the three or four items your child can choose from, and then let the child make the decision. Remember to stay away from deep fried foods. Most restaurants will make a dish to order so request foods that are baked or broiled if they are not on the menu. Remember to include lots of vegetables with dinner. Since many restaurants serve such large portions, be prepared to take home the leftovers for a healthy dinner another night! If your family likes Chinese food, just avoid any deep fried dishes and stick with those that are steamed or sautéed. Request brown rice instead of white rice, and pass on those deep fried noodles that are often served at the beginning of the meal. Even fast food restaurants almost always offer grilled foods. Stay away from the French fries and opt for salads with a limited amount of dressing.

ANTICIPATE includes developing an exercise habit. It is very important for children to get into the habit of exercising every day. Exercising should be as automatic as daily bathing. Take a small amount of time during the day and start to exercise with your children. It is important for the child to know it is "exercise time." This will instill an enduring habit. You can use the exercises on the Next Generation Fitness DVD, or develop your own routine for you and your family. Take five or ten minutes to start your day with stretches, push-ups, squat thrusts and sit-ups.

Children as young as 3 years old should start to develop exercise habits. Even children younger than 3 will benefit from observing their family members engaging in healthy activities and may even want to join in. When my daughter was very young, my husband and I would take her with us to the jogging track. We would alternate jogging around the track and she would stay and play with the other parent. One day she decided she wanted to try and jog with me around the track. I thought it was cute and figured she would stop after about 30 seconds. To my utter surprise, she completed one complete lap around the track! No matter how much I told her to stop, she wanted to "run like mommy." She was just under 3 years old at the time, but she was not even winded. Children are truly amazing!

Eliminate

It is very important to make sure that everyone in the family has healthy eating habits so this next step is particularly crucial. Elimination means the *whole family* must be eating **only** healthy food choices; empty calorie food choices should **not** be kept in the house. The Next Generation Fitness Program will never work if one family member has a restricted diet, regardless of the reason—on a "diet," "watching his or her weight," or even "healthy eating"—while unhealthy foods are available for everyone else in the household.

When I talk to parents about eliminating non-nutritious foods from their household, a common response is concern about "depriving" their child. I generally remind the parent that by allowing their child to have foods like ice cream and donuts all the time, they actually are depriving their child of something: good nutrition and a healthy start to life. In addition, unhealthy eating causes much more long-term damage than can be compensated by a few minutes of taste satisfaction.[2] Allowing your child to think that is it okay to eat high-fat, non-nutritious foods every day is the kind of thinking that has helped bring about the obesity epidemic. It's time to change that thinking. Visualize you and your child aging together! But that image is marred if you are enjoying your later years while your child is encountering health problems and is aging at a faster rate than you are, essentially catching up to you in years. The good news is that we can prevent this fate. However, be clear that it will happen if you let your child eat non-nutrient filled foods and avoid exercising regularly.[3]

Elimination of all unhealthy food from the household is critical to the success of changing your family's lifestyle habits for the better. The Next Generation Fitness Program will fail if it is presented as a special "diet" program for one child who needs to lose weight and not all family members are involved. If the other members of the household are allowed to eat non-nutritious foods and/or junk foods, the "diet" will be perceived as nothing more than discrimination. Anger and resentment will be inevitable and can only result in disharmony in the family. If junk foods and other empty calorie choices are not in the house, it eliminates this conflict. When you are hungry, poor food choices simply aren't available.

It is interesting to note that children who are raised on healthy foods do not seem to crave sweets and other unhealthy foods. The junk-food lifestyle leads to craving more junk food; the more we eat, the more we want. Since sugar is such a major ingredient in the sweets we love and crave in some junk foods, it is important to understand why it is a problem. First, our body needs sugar to supply the energy for cellular functions. The question is how much and what kind of sugar. There are several different kinds of sugar. *Glucose* is the sugar that our body relies on as its primary fuel, so when we eat foods that contain sugar, the body goes into action to process it and break it down into glucose and absorb it into the bloodstream.

Many foods have a natural sugar content, for example fructose, the sugar in fruits, or lactose, the sugar in milk. These sugars are what we call simple sugars and they generally are absorbed into the body quickly because they do not need a lot of processing to convert to glucose. The blood level of glucose rises and falls depending on both the quantity and kind of sugars we ingest. The blood level of glucose must stay within a certain range for healthy functioning.

Foods that contain high amounts of sucrose (table sugar) cause abnormal responses from the hormones that regulate appetite and blood sugar. When we ingest sucrose or high fructose corn syrup, the glucose level in the blood rises higher and more rapidly than it does with fructose alone or other complex carbohydrates like high fiber cereal. We are starting to learn more and more about the body's response to high fructose corn syrup, which is used in a surprising number of processed foods and is often used in place of sucrose. This is not to be confused with the fructose in fruits. High fructose corn syrup contains large amounts of fructose combined with glucose, and this combination causes a quick, elevated rise in blood sugar setting off hormonal responses that increase fat cell mass, appetite and obesity.[4] When the body responds with rapid swings in blood sugar, the urge to eat is so strong that we often will overeat.[5] When eating a well-balanced diet filled with fiber, the glucose level rises slowly. These sugar highs and lows do not occur and the food cravings disappear. Healthy food choices are more satisfying and filling because they contain fiber and of course will promote a healthier life for you and your family.

The effect of sugars on the hormonal responses explains a lot about how we feel after eating certain foods.[6] If we ELIMINATE the junk foods from the household and our diet, we will also eliminate the blood sugar highs and lows. The food cravings for sweets decrease, and eating well just becomes easier. It is a cycle that is self-perpetuating: keep eating well and you will only want to eat well. If you suddenly start to eat high-sugar foods after eating a well-balanced diet for a few weeks you will **feel** the difference. You will feel sluggish and weak and will lack energy. The change is so obvious that you will naturally avoid eating a high-sugar diet.[7]

The sugar cycle also affects children and can even cause mood swings. Parents will often tell me that their child is irritable or moody but they don't attribute this to the child's diet. One parent came to me in tears because she thought her child must have a serious physical ailment. The child had recently become very irritable and had temper outbursts that he had never had before. I examined the child and could find no obvious cause. I started to ask questions about the child's diet and discovered that his diet consisted mainly of bagels and sugary cereals; he refused to eat any meats, fruits or vegetables. His body's response to this horrible diet was swings in blood sugar that translated into constant irritability. Once the poor food choices were eliminated from the household, the child had no choice but to eat the foods made available to him. Although this transition did take time (and some frantic phone calls to me), the child is now on the right track. His mood swings have disappeared and he is on a path to a healthier life.

As parents, we are responsible for everything our child puts into his or her body. We are generally careful about watching babies to make sure they don't put non-food objects in their mouths. I have received numerous phone calls about children who have swallowed something like a piece of a plastic wrapper. I reassure the frantic parent that if the child has already swallowed it without choking, the plastic is usually harmless. We need to train ourselves to think similarly about the harm done to our children when they ingest unhealthy foods. Unhealthy foods have serious consequences. Yet we don't react the same way. If you give in to your child's food cravings, it is no different from allowing your child to eat potentially harmful non-food items. By eliminating these options from the household, you regain control. Try to ignore the whining, the unrealistic fear that you are "starving your child" and the guilt. Think only of your child's well-being.

If we have eliminated the option of having junk foods at home, eating at home is always healthy and nutritious. But we must also recognize the reality of the world we live in and strike a balance. When you are out of the house, do not **completely** restrict treats. This will give your child the benefit of having a great nutritional intake while also allowing for occasional indulgences. Placing extreme limitations on foods, however, can be counterproductive. Children who are never allowed to have sweets often wind up sneaking the forbidden foods and making the problem worse. Sweets and other unhealthy foods shouldn't be taboo; they should merely be limited. It is always better to present things in a positive light. Remind your child about the benefits of all the healthy foods and why it is important that we eat them.

Of course families who eat out every night need to treat these meals as they would meals at home and keep their indulgence in sweets and unhealthy foods to a minimum. Remember that if you are eating well-balanced, nutrient-dense foods, you are not likely to crave unhealthy foods. You will see a difference in yourself and your family. The "temptation" of eating cookies, candies and cakes will decrease while the enjoyment of healthy eating will bring you new-found energy and a feeling of well-being.

We also need to apply the ELIMINATE principle to exercise: We need to ELIMINATE bad habits; we need to ELIMINATE allowing our children long hours of TV, videogames and computer use. As with foods, parents must set limits on these sedentary activities and encourage more physical activity, including exercise.

I was giving a lecture to an audience of parents on instilling healthy habits in children and was asked how to handle a 5-year-old child who consistently chose TV watching over active outdoor play with his father. The father said ruefully, "I wish I could get him to stop watching TV." I told the father that he was forgetting who actually had control of the TV; he could simply turn it off. The father was understandably concerned about starting a battle with his son. Instead of taking charge of the situation, this very good father let his son decide that it was okay to watch TV whenever he wanted. Once you have set a limit to the TV time, of course, you can't force participation in some activity of your choosing. This father couldn't force his son to play ball with him, but he certainly could tell him no more TV. Children learn best when parents set examples, set limits and offer healthy options.

Educate

Once parents understand the concepts of a healthy lifestyle, they need to EDUCATE their children about food and how good food choices help their bodies. As soon as children are old enough, we should describe to them the benefits of eating fruits and vegetables in as much detail as they can understand, and we should do this on a regular basis. Young children believe everything a parent says and if you tell your children about the benefits of foods, they will absorb this information eagerly. The earlier they learn about healthy food facts, the more likely that eating healthy will become second nature to them.

When children are a little older, you can explain to them in simple terms that some foods have many more healthy molecules than others. You can also use visualization techniques with them: Have them draw a mental picture of healthy foods acting like soldiers protecting their hearts and brains. Or they can visualize themselves wearing a suit of armor, protecting them from the unhealthy molecules in junk foods. Explain that food nutrients act in the same way to protect them. Be creative and make these discussions fun.

Children of all ages should also learn about the detrimental effects of unhealthy foods so that they understand why some foods are poor choices. Even very young children will get your message if you use age-appropriate language. For example, simply stating that a particular food is not good for your body will be sufficient information for the younger child. When your child is old enough to understand more complex concepts, tell him or her why certain foods should be avoided; describe the possible damaging effects that the repeated ingestion of a high-fat, low fruit and vegetable diet will have on the body. Have them visualize the body as a tin can, left exposed to the elements where it decays and rusts. A body that is not protected by phytonutrients will also be more likely to "decay" when chronically exposed to a high-saturated fat, nutrient-deficient diet.

The older child can naturally absorb more complicated information and will want to know more. As your child gets older, you can be more specific about why a particular food is not healthy and even include information about free radicals and antioxidants. Help your child visualize the free radicals doing damage inside of the body. Many children have no idea that food could possibly cause damage to their bodies on a molecular level. In my talks with adolescent patients, I have found that many of them know molecular chemistry in great detail, but don't know how foods and free radicals affect them! They usually listen very intently when I explain the concept. I can only influence children one check-up at a time, but as parents we can affect generations of children.

Adults generally are informed about the benefits of exercising, but children need to be taught. When children are out playing, praise them for keeping healthy. Tell them about how they are working their muscles and keeping their bones strong. Keep this statement simple for the younger children, but with older children and adolescents, talk to them about heart disease and blood pressure. Children are very smart and get the connection between being active and keeping a healthy heart. When giving a lecture to a class of first graders on "heart health," I was amazed at the questions that these young children came up with. It was clear that they absolutely understood the concept of the heart as a muscle that needs to be exercised every day. They were fascinated by the subject and could not get enough information. They wanted to know what foods to eat and how much exercise they should get. They even told me that smoking was bad for the heart!

Participate

The whole family **must** PARTICIPATE in the Next Generation Fitness Program to ensure its success. The old adage "do as I say, not as I do" is applicable when trying to teach your children about healthy lifestyles. Children are much more likely to follow your lead if you set the example. Just talking about proper foods and exercise and asking children to follow the plan is not enough; you have to be engaged in it, too. If you are having trouble following a healthy lifestyle, visualize the benefits of good health for your loved ones as well as yourself.

Like it or not, you are a role model for your child and it is the most important job that you will have as a parent. It is easy to see how we unconsciously influence our children; we see our children pick up certain expressions that we use, imitate our body movements or even use our voice inflections. The impact we have on our offspring is never ending and we must try to be the best role models possible.

It is natural for all young children to want to be like their parents. Parents can be assured that when their children are young, they will follow the lead of their parents. As children get older, however, they become more independent and are more likely to rebel and do the opposite of what their parents do or what their parents want them to do. Adolescence is a time when teens want to learn for themselves, try to establish independence and experiment with making their own decisions. This is just the nature of adolescence. So if you have not already formed healthy habits in your children's daily routines by the time they are teens, it won't be an easy thing to do. However, this doesn't mean you shouldn't try; maintaining a healthy diet for both you and your family will always have positive results. Bringing healthy changes into a household while including your adolescents will only have a positive impact on them. They may be resistant to changes, and anything you say may only result in a roll of the eyes. But continue to follow the plan and only good things will come.

We also need to remember the exercise component. Exercising with children even when they are very young is an important part of the Next Generation Fitness Program. It is never too early to expose little ones to exercise. Mothers who are trying to get back into shape after pregnancy can take their babies to exercise classes and even be creative with play time by exercising with the baby. There are so many ways to expose your children to physical activity and ensure that they learn about the benefits of exercising. If parents get their children into the **habit** of exercising while they are young, it is a gift that will last a lifetime. The goal is healthy eating and exercise habits that stay with your family for life.

If your family has been eating poorly for years and your children are already pre-adolescents or even adolescents, it may be easier to start to change to a healthier lifestyle one step at a time. Start by planning only healthy choices for breakfast. As time goes on, make only healthy choices for dinner and start to ELIMINATE junk food desserts. If your family is not used to healthy eating, you might hear some complaining. Ignore it and continue to plan meals that are best for your family's health. Then start to plan some family exercise time. This will be a big shock if nobody likes to exercise. Start by using the Next Generation Fitness DVD, or just get them up and moving around; go for family walks, hikes or bike rides. Even running up and down the stairs a few times is a great start. Everything can be done slowly and in small bite-size pieces.

Once you have been giving your family healthy meal choices for a few weeks (or even months if it takes that long to get everyone comfortable with them), remove the junk foods from the household and replace them with healthy snacks. *(See Recipes section for additional ideas, p. 115.)* You can even move slowly on this step by gradually replacing junk food snacks like chips with baked crackers; then replace the cookies with frozen yogurt. Continue with this kind of swapping until fruit is the number one sweet treat in the house!

EDUCATE your family slowly as you make each change. Explain the reason for the specific changes so that they too understand about nutrients, heart-healthy foods, a longer life, etc. Use whatever language is appropriate for the age of your children. You want them to understand that your reason for taking away

the French fries is a legitimate one. Of course, you will be participating with the rest of your family; no family can maximize the
health of their children if the parents are not willing to live a
healthy lifestyle too. I will never forget a consult in which I was
asked to advise a family on how to become healthy eaters. After
an hour and a half discussion of all the foods the family needed
to eat and the type of exercises they needed to do, the three
children were very eager and excited about getting started. The
father turned to me and announced that he could do the exercises and start to eat fruit, but he would never "touch a vegetable." The children asked the obvious question: why did they
have to eat vegetables if their father did not? The father did not
realize that by stating categorically that he would not eat vegetables, his children would never do it either! We always must
remember that our children emulate our behavior.

Questions & Answers

1

Q) I have not tried the program yet and I am
concerned because my children already have
poor eating habits. It seems impossible to get
them to eat vegetables, so how am I supposed to
get them to eat well?

A) This is a very common problem, but one that can be solved
with patience, commitment and persistence. If you have been
following the steps in *Growing Up Healthy* (ANTICIPATE,
ELIMINATE, EDUCATE and PARTICIPATE), your child will
naturally have good eating habits. Parents who had good health
habits prior to having children, probably were unaware that
they were already using the steps outlined in this program to
ensure healthy eating in their children.

If your child already has poor eating habits, it indicates that you missed the ANTICIPATE step as well as the ELIMINATE step. This is common so don't worry. You can still be successful with the Next Generation Fitness Program. As discussed in the ANTICIPATE step, think about meals ahead of time and plan for healthy ones. Then follow the ELIMINATE step by getting rid of all junk food in the house and frequenting only restaurants that offer healthy choices. *(For more details about these steps and how to handle approaching them with your family, see ANTICIPATE, p. 24 and ELIMINATE, p. 30.)* Setting limits is an integral part of parenting and needs to be applied to eating and dietary habits. If eating out is an occasional treat, you can allow your child more freedom with the choices. But if you are always eating out, you need to set limitations when in a restaurant. Find restaurants that have healthy choices. It's not as difficult as you think. Many restaurants are beginning to recognize the market for healthier menu choices, and as the demand grows, so will these kinds of menus.

2

Q) **I give my kindergartner a healthy snack for school everyday, but she eats other children's snacks that are non-nutritious. What do I do?**

A) If you encounter a problem like this, you must talk to your child's teacher. This should not happen in a kindergarten while there is a teacher in the room. The teacher is responsible for everything that goes on in the class and needs to make sure children are not exchanging food, especially because of the danger posed by food allergies. Try to enlist the support of your child's teacher in discouraging unhealthy snacks. Teachers have a tremendous impact on children and if they start out the school year reminding the children to bring in only healthy snacks, chances are the children will follow their direction. If possible, try to get the whole school on board. Parents can also make some snack recommendations that are healthy and fun and can be shared with the other parents. If your child's school reinforces the healthy habits you are fostering at home, it will make your job that much easier.

3

Q) When my child refuses to eat what I have made for dinner, should I prepare something else?

A) This is a very common problem within families today. Parents tend to cater to their children by preparing different meals or even purchasing different fast foods to satisfy everyone at the table. Instead, we need to make one meal with two or three choices—for example broccoli, sweet potato and chicken. If your child refuses all of these choices, then he or she is not hungry enough to eat. Do not make a special meal for the child who refuses to eat! But do not make it a battle either. Simply remind your child that this is dinner and there are three choices; the child can eat any one or more of these choices. Be clear that if the child is not hungry, he or she does not have to eat. NEVER force your child to eat or clean the plate. If this ever becomes a battle, it is one that you will never win, and it could backfire by turning into an eating disorder.

4

Q) What if my child refuses to eat what I have made but is willing and able to prepare a healthy alternative?

A) This is an acceptable situation. If your child is old enough and willing to prepare a healthy food choice, there is no reason to stop him or her. However, when children are younger, it sends a negative signal if you prepare more than one meal. Do not worry if children go to bed without eating. A common fear among parents is that if their child goes to bed without eating, something terrible will happen. This leads to so much parental anxiety that parents will give their child a non-nutrient-dense choice rather than no food at all. Parents need to stop this behavior. A hungry child will eat most foods; just make sure that they are healthy ones. Thankfully, most of us in the U.S. and other developed nations are not faced with starvation, so there is no reason to worry that your child will starve. In fact, the child who goes to bed without dinner will wake up all the more hungry in the morning; in a healthy choice household, the child will eat a good breakfast!

5

Q) **When I buy fresh fruits and vegetables for the family to snack on, I often end up throwing some of the food away because it has spoiled. How can I encourage the family to eat these foods?**

A) We have all gone through this with our families. The kids are complaining that there is nothing to eat, but the fridge is filled with strawberries, peppers and blueberries! Make healthy food choices easily available and ready to eat, and everyone in the household will do just that–eat them. Keep the fresh fruit washed and ready to eat. Cut the vegetables up and keep them where the family can see them when the fridge is open. It needs to be right in front of their eyes and ready to eat!

6

Q) **What are some healthy snack suggestions for my child who is always on the go?**

A) Some of the best foods are very portable. Nuts are my number one favorite healthy snack. They are loaded with nutrition and packed with energy. Be careful about eating too many because they do contain a lot of fat, even though it's the "good" kind of fat. Fruits are also a very convenient snack, and there are many to choose from. They are all loaded with nutrients and energy. Dried fruit is also a good snack, but watch for added sugar and preservatives. Olives are a little thought of snack, but again are packed with energy and nutrition. (Olives contain a lot of salt so limit this choice.) High-fiber cereal in a sealed plastic bag is another perfectly fine, portable snack; it needs no refrigeration and will keep for a long time. Air-popped popcorn is also a great snack. Make sure it is air-popped and not loaded with butter.

7

Q) My daughter uses her allowance money to buy junk foods and candy at school. How can I discourage this behavior?

A) Remember, you are in charge. Be very specific about how allowance money may be used. Most elementary-school-age children do not need to bring money to school. If you do let your child buy a snack each day, tell her the choices that she is allowed to have, but be prepared if she does not follow your advice. There is a lot of peer pressure in school even when it comes to eating. I have a young patient who has been monitored for weight for the past year. One of the problems is the peer pressure she encounters in the school cafeteria where they serve fried chicken, ice cream, chips and sodas. Her peers were not trying to be mean; they wanted their friend to eat the same foods as they did. My patient and I had a long discussion about how the other children were not being taught good nutrition and how she was much more knowledgeable about healthy food choices. She became empowered by her superior knowledge.

If you find that your child is spending money everyday on junk foods in school, you can remove the privilege of allowing the child to buy the snack; your daughter can then bring a healthy snack from home. Her allowance money may then be used elsewhere.

8

Q) How do I handle it when every time my son goes to his best friend's house, he fills himself with junk food?

A) This situation is easily handled. Most children who have healthy eating habits will tend to avoid gorging themselves because they know it will make them feel physically unwell. The child who is looking for the opportunity to eat junk every time he is out of the house needs to be reminded about the health benefits of eating well and the detrimental effects of eating poorly.

Talk with the parents of your son's friend and ask them to refrain from making these food choices available to your son. You would insist that they do the same if your child was nut-allergic. You could offer to have your child bring his own snack to their home. This has happened to me in the reverse. My son has a friend who loves soda and would ask for it whenever he visited. Since soda is not one of the drink choices in my household, he had to "suffer" with orange juice or water. One day he was invited over for a holiday dinner and he brought two cans of Dr Pepper with him. I could only laugh and remind him of the poor choices he was making. As a pediatrician, it is very hard for me to watch children make such poor choices so I feel compelled to say things (much to my children's dismay). I try never to make it demeaning or sound like a lecture and to keep it light and humorous.

9

Q) How is it possible for me to get my children to exercise when they have never expressed any desire to do so in the past.

A) EDUCATE and PARTICIPATE. Teach your children about all the advantages that exercising will give them, from running faster, jumping higher, being stronger and even doing better in school. Show your children that you are exercising, too, and share with them the benefits you get from exercising. Explain this in concrete terms and tell them how the exercise makes you feel physically. The impact that adults have on kids is amazing. When my youngest child's friends come over and see me working out, most of them ask me to show them how to do the exercise and they want to start to exercise in their homes as well. Show them and they will follow.

10

Q) What types of foods should I offer my child when he is sick? If he doesn't feel well enough to eat, should I force the situation?

A) Good nutrition is important all the time, and even more so when a child is ill and the body needs to fight and recover. Children commonly loose their appetite when they are ill. Don't force solid foods, but offer the same healthy choices. However, you must make sure that your child drinks plenty of liquids so he does not dehydrate. I often recommend smoothie drinks with fruits, nuts and milk. You can pack nutrition into a smoothie, satisfy the liquid requirement, avoid a food battle and stave off dehydration. The only caveat is if your child is vomiting and/or has diarrhea, in which case you need to rehydrate him. Consult with your pediatrician on what is best for your child.

chapter four

Foods That Children Should Eat & What Makes Them Special!

It is such a pleasure to see children eating healthy foods! Every parent needs continual reminders about how certain foods can cause disease, and, more importantly, how other foods can prevent disease. Use visualizations to reinforce these concepts for yourself and help your children to do the same.

Following is a list of some of the more nutritious foods that children tend to avoid. Of course not every child refuses to eat these foods, but from my observations over the many years that I have been in practice, these foods are the least likely to be on a child's menu. However, these foods can make an outstanding contribution to our health. If we could make sure that our children eat one or more of these foods every day, we could be adding years to their lives.

FATTY FISH

This category includes salmon, mackerel, tuna and sardines. These fish in particular contain essential omega-3 fatty acids. These fatty acids are not produced in the body but they are required for proper body functioning. Our body takes omega-3 fatty acids and uses them to make other molecules that inhibit platelet aggregation and decrease inflammation inside the body. We need to eat these foods on a regular basis to assure that we get a good supply of omega-3 fatty acids.[1]

Studies have shown that a diet rich in these essential fatty acids will dramatically decrease the risk of sudden death from heart disease, decrease blood triglycerides (fats) and protect against heart disease and hypertension.[2] Some other major advantages of omega-3 fatty acids include protection against memory loss, age-related loss of cognitive function and depression; research indicates that these fatty acids may even stave off dementia.[3] Omega-3 fatty acids are also very important in early fetal development of the brain and eyes.[4]

Children generally do not get enough of these essential fatty acids and as a result, they may manifest some minor symptoms of deficiency. These symptoms include increased anxiety, depression, decreased ability to concentrate, menstrual cramps and irritability. You may notice these symptoms in your child and not think they are related to diet. Try increasing the omega-3 fatty acid content in your child's daily diet. You can do this by serving fatty fish twice a week and using flax meal or walnuts daily. If your child has had a limited amount of these foods in the past and then starts to eat them on a daily basis, you are likely to see some minor changes in the child's behavior—increased energy and decreased irritability. Often these changes will be noticeable within six months. You may also notice some improvement in your child's school work because these foods enhance the ability to concentrate, resulting in less frustration and more positive emotional energy.

Note that if you eat salmon, try to eat fresh rather than farm-raised salmon. The farm-raised salmon have an unacceptably high level of environmental contaminants.[5] Other foods that contain omega-3 fatty acids include walnuts, eggs yolks from chickens that have been fed foods with omega-3 fatty acids in them, green leafy vegetables and flaxseeds or flax meal. Adding omega-3-rich foods to your child's diet will have a tremendously positive impact on his or her health. There is such a variety of foods that contain these substances that it is easy to ensure that your child gets them regularly. If your child hates fish, there are still the other options—so no excuses! *(See Recipes section, p. 115, for some suggestions.)*

There is no current recommendation on the amount of omega-3 fatty acids for children although the American Heart Association and other medical agencies have issued recommendations for adult intake.

SPINACH, KALE, PEPPERS, KIWI FRUIT & RED GRAPES

These foods have a very high content of lutein and zeaxanthin, both powerful antioxidants. Because these foods, in particular, contain such a powerhouse of antioxidants, they can snuff out the free radicals that cause such tremendous damage inside our bodies if they are not neutralized.[6] Many diseases cause an increase in the production of free radicals and eating these foods can help combat them. It has been shown that lutein and zeaxanthin can dissolve into the eyes and act as powerful antioxidants to protect the inside of our eyes.[7] The protection afforded by these nutrients decreases the risk of cataract development and age-related decline in vision. Children suffering with diseases like diabetes will especially benefit from these powerhouse foods because the disease produces more free radicals, which often cause an increased incidence of eye disease.

CRUCIFEROUS VEGETABLES

These vegetables include broccoli, broccolini, kale, chard, cauliflower, brussels sprouts and cabbage. These vegetables all contain large amounts of phytonutrients that have very potent anticancer properties.[8] Broccolini is particularly rich in these cancer-fighting nutrients.[9] Every day your child should have a vegetable from this category of foods. You will be doing a great service for your children if you help them get in the habit of eating one of these vegetables on a regular basis.

ONIONS & GARLIC

These two foods are so common that we hardly think of them as health foods. Little do most people know that they are packed with disease-fighting nutrients.[10] Parents often ask me what they can do to prevent their children from getting sick or how they can help them get better when they are sick. I always tell parents to make sure their children eat lots of fruits and vegetables even when they are sick and to use lots of garlic and onions in their cooking! Most parents are amazed when I mention garlic because they don't realize its healing powers. To get children to eat garlic, I advise parents to simply add a little fresh raw or lightly cooked garlic to the child's favorite dinner foods. Parents have always been grateful for this tidbit and have never come back to me saying their child refused to eat their favorite food with garlic in it!

Onions and garlic are often added as seasoning to many recipes and are easy to include in your child's diet. The phytonutrients that make onions and garlic so special are organosulfur compounds, which can decrease the risk of gastrointestinal and prostate cancers.[11] Eating onions and garlic, even in small quantities, will cause platelets to become less sticky; sticky platelets are a factor in increased risk of stroke. Onions and garlic also stimulate the immune system because the organosulfur compounds have antibacterial and antioxidant capabilities.[12]

GRAPEFRUIT

This fruit is usually passed up by children and often thought to be too much trouble for adults to eat. Let me give you several reasons why you should put grapefruit on your shopping list on a regular basis. First of all, grapefruit ingestion will activate your body's own defense system to fend off those nasty free radicals. In addition, grapefruit helps increase new bone formation, protect our DNA against damage from radiation and inhibit the growth of human tumor cells.[13] Grapefruit also has a positive effect on sugar metabolism by helping your body use glucose more efficiently.[14] Eating grapefruit regularly will also help lower your cholesterol levels![15]

Have I convinced you to eat grapefruit yet? The phytonutrient naringin is the special compound in grapefruit that gives it all the wonderful aforementioned qualities. Grapefruit has a substantial amount of naringin—more than that found in other citrus fruits—and there are few phytonutrients that can rival its protective effects. Eating naringin-containing foods daily can have life-altering affects on your child's future. Visualize those nutrients charging up your child's defense system to protect against the free radicals that are formed from living and breathing. Think of the nutrients killing off the potential cancer cells that our body makes regularly. Our body does indeed make cells that can become cancerous, but we have a natural defense system that destroys these cells before they can become a problem; naringin aides this system and helps to keep us free from cancer. With all these benefits, why wouldn't you have this fruit in your house and encourage everyone to eat it?

Although grapefruit may be a magic fruit in terms of health prevention there is a caveat. There are specific compounds in the grapefruit that can inhibit the metabolism of certain drugs. For anyone taking prescription medications, be sure to ask your doctor about eating grapefruit while you are taking the medication. This does not diminish the great benefits of the fruit and it is not a reason to cross it off your shopping list. But it is a reminder that there are always some foods and drugs that may have negative interactions.

SOYBEANS & TOFU

Soybeans have long been a staple in Asian culture and we have been able to learn a lot about the benefits of soy products by studying these populations.[16] What we have learned may be enough to convince even the most persistent soybean antagonist to start to enjoy them!

The American Heart Association has allowed soy foods to include the organization's stamp of approval as a heart healthy food. This was permitted because some studies indicate that eating soy products reduces cholesterol. However, the data is inconclusive.[17] More studies need to be done to elucidate the cholesterol and soy health link. This is NOT the reason I think soy products should be included in a child's diet. Soy contains compounds called isoflavones and these compounds can mimic or inhibit the effect of estrogen in our bodies and act as antioxidants.[18] This effect produces a myriad of benefits. To start with, soy consumption may decrease the incidence of breast, uterine and prostate cancers.[19] It also seems to have a positive effect on bone density thereby decreasing the risk of osteoporosis in later years. Because soy contains antioxidants, it will also decrease heart disease and inhibit clogging of the arteries.[20]

Using tofu in foods for children is so easy because tofu absorbs the taste of the food you mix it with; it is easily mixed into fruit shakes, soups and dips. Many families use soy products on a regular basis without realizing the benefits of using them. Soy products are high in protein and provide essential amino acids, which are the building blocks for proteins. In addition, soy products can provide an alternative to high-saturated-fat meats, another benefit, especially for those who have high cholesterol.

GREEN TEA

We generally do not think of tea as a health food; however, green tea is loaded with phytonutrients that are unsurpassed in their antioxidant abilities.[21] Parents generally avoid giving their children tea or coffee mainly out of concern about the caffeine content. What most of us don't realize is that chocolate and most sodas have as much or more caffeine per serving than a small cup of green tea. Parents may fear that caffeine will stunt growth, but this is not true. The phytonutrients in green tea have anti-aging (protects against sun damage!), antioxidant and anticancer properties. It is thought that green tea is the answer to what is known as the Asian paradox:[22] Some Asian countries have very high tobacco usage but low rates of heart disease and lung cancer. Research on this data is slowly showing the protective factor to be the antioxidants in green tea. Put green tea on your menu!

chapter five

The Plan

Being aware of the obesity epidemic and its causes, knowing how to change our thinking about nutrition and exercise and taking the steps needed to solve the problems are all important parts of making healthy and positive changes to our lifestyle. Now we will look at the specifics of the Next Generation Fitness Program: the process of planning and goal setting, the foods that are best to include in our family's diets and the best type of exercises for children.

The Next Generation Fitness Program will help you achieve lifelong good health through a nutrition plan that should last a lifetime and an exercise program that can be practiced anywhere. Lifelong good heath requires planning and we need to plan carefully so we can maximize our nutrient intake. With the Next Generation Fitness Program, this goal is easily attainable. Following this program will increase longevity and decrease your risk for heart disease, some cancers, stroke, high blood pressure, type II diabetes and possibly Alzheimer's disease.

Planning and goal setting are important for all aspects of our lives but it seems like when it comes to diet and exercise, we just don't make them priorities. Most of us are already short on time and long on lists of things to do. As a result, we don't spend enough time planning for our daily nutrition so we don't anticipate our nutritional needs on a daily basis. For example, when we get out of bed in the morning and go into the kitchen to grab a bite to eat, we haven't usually planned what we are going to eat. We just eat what is available at that particular time. For most people, the same behavior applies to lunch. If you bring a bagged lunch to school or work, you or someone else took some time to plan that meal. If you buy lunch without a nutrition plan in mind, the only plan is what the store or restaurant offers and depending on the venue, you may be dramatically limiting your healthy food choices. Unfortunately, the same limitation can apply to dinner. But meal planning is very important. We need to put some thought into not only what we are eating, but also what we are going to eat at the next meal. Everything requires planning if you are going to achieve your goal.

Next Generation Fitness is a family-based program designed to improve the overall health of anyone who follows it. It is essential for parents to engage in the program with their children. Proper nutrition and exercise are habits that must be modeled, taught and incorporated into our lifestyle; they cannot be dictated. Parents need to work side-by-side with their children to plan meals, exercise and be a life coach. Once your family becomes familiar with the nutrition and the exercise components of the program, they will start to become healthy habits. Once habits are formed, less planning is needed because habits are automatic and don't require much conscious thought; at that point the Next Generation Fitness Program will be an integral part of your life.

Understanding the Nutrient Value of Foods

A great nutrition plan involves eating a lot of low-calorie, nutrient-dense foods. Nutrient-dense foods are foods that are filled with nutrients but not filled with calories. Unfortunately, as we have seen, the trend is for more and more people to move away from good eating and toward consuming more calorie-dense, nutrient-deficient processed foods. The results are devastating, obvious and completely preventable. Anticipating these results will help avoid the problem. The main foods recommended in the Next Generation Fitness Program were chosen because of their nutrient value—they are all nutrient-dense and have phytonutrients that will help prevent many diseases.

In most families there is little emphasis on the family meal with healthy choices. As a result, children today are consuming processed foods on a regular basis. Every day, they are eating chips, cakes, cookies, donuts, ice cream, candy, and/or chocolate. I spend a lot of time in my office trying to convince parents of the importance of their child's food intake. Many parents mistakenly believe that if their children already eat fruits, vegetables and meats, it is okay to for them to also have chips or ice cream every day, whether as a dessert or as a reward for good eating. This is not a good practice for many reasons. First, parents should never use one food to bribe a child to eat another food. This could backfire and create an eating disorder by giving the child control over something that is a goal of the parent. Giving a child the power to manipulate a situation on a daily basis is a dangerous thing. Furthermore, our children don't need the extra saturated fat that is contained in most desserts. Offering fruit as a dessert provides so much more nutrition. Also remember that if you have sweets and junk foods in the house, you are breaking the ELIMINATE rule and it will be counterproductive. The rationale that accompanies this thinking needs to change; it is not okay to have these types of foods in the household. If you don't follow all the steps, including ELIMINATE, you will not be successful.

As we saw earlier, free radicals can cause extensive damage inside the body, and eating junk foods increases the production of free radicals, causes excess calorie consumption and offers no benefits from nutrients and antioxidants. An excess of free radicals can put your body into an oxidative stress state, leaving you vulnerable to heart disease, stroke, increased cancer risk and possible dementia. And of course junk foods also increase the risk of obesity with all the inherent problems of that condition: hypertension; arthritis; type II diabetes, which then can cause kidney failure; blindness; loss of limb, and more. Do I need to give you more reasons to avoid eating junk food on a regular basis? Start setting some nutritional goals for you and your family.

Remember that the calories from foods that we eat need to be converted into energy. Energy is made available to our cells by using a multitude of enzymes, vitamins and minerals. There are hundreds of chemical reactions that are required to convert food sources (fats, carbohydrates, proteins) into usable energy. Without the proper cofactors in the form of vitamins and minerals, these reactions will not take place efficiently. Choosing foods that are not full of these nutrients may put the body at risk. Foods like soda, cake, cookies, candy, most fast foods, juice drinks and chips are nutritionally deficient. They offer empty calories— calories with very few if any of the accompanying essential vitamins, minerals and phytonutrients needed by the body. If we consume an excess of calories, the body will always convert them into fat, regardless of the food source, and the fats will be stored in the body, causing a weight gain. This occurs no matter what kind of food you eat. So if you have been eating more calories than your body is burning, even if all the calories came from protein, your body will still store the excess as fat.

Each food that we eat contributes something to our body. Every cell in our body is like a factory that needs hundreds of workers to keep it running. Those workers include vitamins, minerals, enzymes and the energy captured from food. Each cell has a specific purpose, like the cardiac cells found only in the heart. These are special muscle cells that are in constant motion and need a constant nutrient supply. If these muscles fail to get the proper nutrition, the results could be serious.

Neurons are the special cells that keep our nervous system (brain and nerve cells throughout the body) running effectively. Neurons allow us to think clearly and make important decisions. These cells contribute to who we are and everything we do. If these cells are deprived of nutrients, the results may be harmful. *The function of neurons is critical to our life, yet most of us never think about what we need to eat to ensure that they are properly nourished every day.* At the cellular level, foods that we eat are used by the body to enable communication between the cells, to keep the cells well nourished and to provide the cells with their protective coating. These actions all contribute to helping the body move and think. One example of the relationship between diet and brain function can be seen when there is a deficiency of vitamin B_{12}. Over a prolonged period of time, this deficiency can lead to neuropsychiatric symptoms.

Neurons need a constant supply of glucose in order to function. If you go to school or work without breakfast, your brain cells are deprived of the glucose they need to function properly. Just like a car that does not have enough gasoline, the cells cannot work well without the proper fuel. Once the supply of glucose is depleted, in order to survive, the body goes into starvation mode and will break down protein from muscles to fuel the brain. Most of us will experience this as feeling tired and not as energetic as usual. Our reflexes will be slower and it becomes harder to concentrate. Since you did not feed your brain, or you fed it nutritionally deficient food, you deprived your cells of the nutrients they needed to utilize the energy for cell work.

Let's compare what happens if you grab a donut or muffin for breakfast rather than a bowl of oatmeal. The donut contains a lot of sugar and will cause a sharper and faster rise in your glucose level than the oatmeal. This higher rise in sugar in turn causes a higher rise in the hormones, like insulin, that act to balance glucose. By mid-morning you will notice that you are not feeling great or you are very hungry because now your body's glucose is starting to drop as rapidly as it rose. A more rapid swing in blood sugar causes a sensation of weakness, a decreased ability to concentrate and an urge to eat. Your brain sensors are telling you to eat because the brain uses glucose as its main fuel and now it's running out of fuel. While grabbing the donut may initially supply your brain with glucose (along with saturated fats, lots of calories and no phytonutrients), later in the morning your body responds as if you had not eaten breakfast at all. Neither option is healthy; both deprived your body of essential nutrients and fuel for daily efficient functioning.

THE DIET MYTH

Diet plans designed for rapid weight loss, in general, are not good for anyone. The many diet plans on the market target people who want to lose weight with quick results. These diets usually only take into account the amount of proteins, carbohydrates and fats that are consumed. I call these 20th-century diets because the developers of these diets do not consider the nutrition information that has been made available in the 21st century. Diets that encourage high-protein or low-carbohydrate intakes are not balanced and cannot be maintained for prolonged periods of time. These diets are often unrealistic and some of them require special foods or meals that have to be purchased. This usually works well for the people who are marketing and selling the diets, but not for those who are trying to follow them.

Dramatically restricting calories or eating unrealistic portions of foods will decrease your metabolic rate and, once you resume your previous eating pattern, not only will you regain the weight, but often you will end up gaining more weight than you lost. In addition to the fact that these diets will most certainly not provide the nutrients you need from foods, they set up a dangerous pattern. The drop in metabolic rate that you experienced while on the diet persists, making it even harder to lose weight the next time you to try to diet again. The cycle continues and you will continue to struggle with weight loss until you make a lifestyle change—a change that will stick with you forever.

Most diet books tell us what we already know: Exercise regularly, eat fruits, vegetables, legumes and whole grains and stay away from foods with trans fats (chemically altered fats), saturated fats and high quantities of processed simple sugars. To lose weight and maintain optimum health, however, a *lifestyle* change needs to be made. *Growing Up Healthy* offers a sophisticated approach by looking at what we are eating to ensure that we get the proper amount of omega-3 fatty acids, carotenoids, bioflavonoids, antioxidants, vitamins, minerals and phytonutrients. The meal plans are designed to help change not only our way of eating, but also the way we think about food and diet, and the exercise plan is designed so that we can continue to exercise regularly for the rest of our lives. These factors contribute to making the change to a healthier life.

chapter six

Daily Nutrition: Balance & Portion Control

The Next Generation Fitness Program includes a nutrition plan that is easy for children to understand and is one that I think will be a welcome change from fad diets and other more mundane nutrition plans. The best and the healthiest nutrition has always been and will remain regularly eating fresh fruits, vegetables, legumes, whole grains, fish and lean meats. Of course you already knew that. If this is the case, why then are we always searching for some panacea that keeps us thin, keeps our skin looking young, staves off disease and increases our energy levels? Although the ideas that form the basis for the Next Generation Fitness Program have been around forever, we still look for a quick fix. This program takes what we have known for decades and adds a new twist so it applies to everyone, including children.

One very important principle of good nutrition is **balance**. Balance involves both variety in the foods we eat and the quantity of food we eat. The Next Generation Fitness plan includes menus that offer variety and flexibility; it also allocates portions so that we can gauge and monitor consumption. The nutrition plan uses a color scheme that represents balance and variety. This color scheme roughly represents the colors of foods, making it easy even for young children to follow and understand. The plan ensures that we eat many different foods each day, providing a maximal intake of phytonutrients. Foods that contain bioflavonoids, carotenoids and other phytonutrients are found mainly in the fruit and vegetable categories. Specifically, certain colored fruits and vegetables contain a larger concentration of certain nutrients. This is why it is so important to include a variety of different colored fruits and vegetables. The color scheme also makes it fun and easy for children to follow. Color identification starts at around the age of 3, which is a good time to make your children "aware" of the food colors and how to follow a good nutrition plan.

We should also note that some nutrition plans encourage eating one type of food in large quantities. This completely ignores the importance of balance. Eating an unbalanced diet will invariably cause problems. For example, low-carbohydrate diets cause the consumption of more protein. The consumption of more protein occurs in order to replace the energy lost by the lack of carbohydrates. This increased protein intake will put stress on your kidneys (protein by-products are excreted in the kidneys) and cause a loss of calcium from your bones. Losing calcium from bones can cause an increase in the risk of getting osteoporosis, a potentially devastating problem.

The other aspect of any nutrition plan is portion control. Americans are eating larger and larger servings of foods, so much so that we have a distorted view of what makes up a serving. Many people think of a serving of pasta as a nice-size bowlful. The truth is that one serving of pasta is one half of a cup—a far cry from that bowl of pasta you had in mind. We need to downsize our portions! Paying attention to serving size is important for everybody. Eating too many calories at *any age* is detrimental. Paying attention to the **amount** of food we eat is a very, very important part of any nutritional plan, and it is an integral part of the Next Generation Fitness Program.

Balance

Good nutrition requires a balance of nutritious foods from each of the basic food groups. The Next Generation Fitness Program uses the color of foods to help you understand what foods your body requires and in what quantities. This system makes the concept easier to remember and more concrete so that children can participate in your menu planning. The food color groups are *Green, Red, Orange, White, Brown, Blue* and *Yellow*. The categories for green, red, orange, blue and yellow include only those fruits and vegetables of the corresponding color. The brown category includes grains and nuts and the white category includes dairy and proteins. It is essential to include each group in your daily meal planning. Foods that contain bioflavonoids, carotenoids and other phytonutrients come mainly from foods in the fruit and vegetable categories. Some color categories of fruits and vegetables contain a larger concentration of specific nutrients than others. This is why it is so important to eat fruits and vegetables from each of the color categories. Each color group contains a wide selection of foods to accommodate many individual taste preferences.

The chart on page 66 uses a puzzle image to illustrate how good nutrition depends on each of the pieces to be complete. Just as a puzzle would be incomplete without all its pieces, the body depends on each of the food groups for specific nutrients. Each of the puzzle pieces roughly represents how much food in each category we should have in our daily diet.

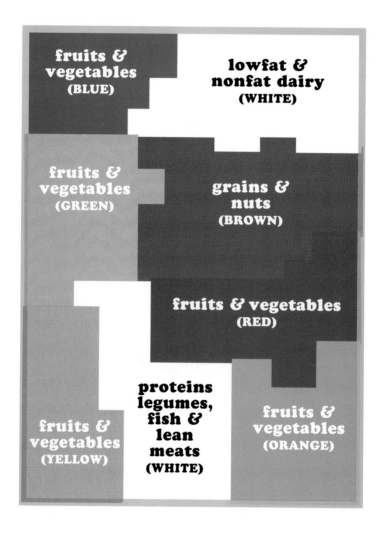

Portion Control

Good nutrition also requires portion control. Eating too much at any age is unhealthy. The portions and recommended servings specified in the meal plans are designed to satisfy hunger and fulfill the phytonutrient requirements for all age groups.

The following simple outline lists each of the basic food groups, some of the foods in each group and the recommended daily requirements for each. The serving sizes are shown for education purposes; we need to understand what constitutes a serving size so we can adjust how our families are eating. The amount of foods and calories children need to eat is mainly dependent on their age, so the recommended servings of foods given in this food list are based on age. When you incorporate this nutrition plan into your daily routine, your child should maintain a steady gain in weight and height (assuming he or she has not attained full growth). If your child is a good weight proportional to height (your pediatrician should tell you if there is concern about weight) and he or she loses weight when you change to healthy eating, you need to increase calorie intake by increasing healthy food choices. People who are overweight and overeat will loose weight when they start to engage in a healthy lifestyle.

BROWN

Grains

ADULTS: start with 6 servings per day from this group, and adjust the number of servings as needed to a maximum of 11 servings.

CHILDREN 3-6 YEARS: 3-4 servings/day
CHILDREN 6-PUBERTY: 4-6 servings/day
ADOLESCENTS: 6-7 servings/day

SERVING SIZE
bread = 1 slice
pasta = 1/2 cup
bagel, bun/roll = 1/2 small size
pita bread = 1/2 small round
tortilla = 1/2 large size
popcorn = 3-4 cups, air-popped
rice = 1/3 cup, cooked
cooked cereal = 1/2 cup dry
cold cereal = 1 ounce
*(Cereal is measured in ounces rather than cups
due to the large variation in weight.)*

Mixed Nuts (raw, roasted)

3 YEARS AND OLDER: 1 serving
SERVING SIZE = 2 tablespoons

GREEN, ORANGE, RED, BLUE & YELLOW

Fruits

ADULTS: 2 - 3 cups/day
CHILDREN 3-6 YEARS: 1 cup/day
CHILDREN 6-PUBERTY: $1^1/2$ cups/day
ADOLESCENTS: $1^1/2$ - $2^1/2$ cups/day

SERVING SIZE
1 medium-sized fruit = 1 cup
8 ounces 100% fruit juice = 1 cup

Mix and match fruits from each of the color categories according to individual taste.

Vegetables

ADULTS: $2^1/2$ - 4 cups/day
CHILDREN 3-6 YEARS: 1 cup/day
CHILDREN 6-PUBERTY: $1^1/2$ - 2 cups/day
ADOLESCENTS: $2^1/2$ - 3 cups/day

SERVING SIZE
1 medium-sized potato = 1 cup of vegetables
2 cups raw leafy greens = 1 cup of vegetables

Select vegetables from any of the color categories when planning your meals. Note that although it is white, cauliflower is included in the green category because it is a vegetable; the white category is reserved for protein-dense foods and dairy products.

WHITE

Protein

ADOLESCENTS AND ADULTS: 2 servings/day,
divided into 2 or 3 meals
CHILDREN 3-PUBERTY: minimum of 1 serving/day
(3 - 4 ounces)

SERVING SIZE
poultry, meat and fish = 3 - 4 ounces
(approximately the size of a deck of cards)
cooked plain beans = 1¹/2 cups
egg whites = 3 - 4 medium eggs
(the egg white contains the protein)
deli meat = 3 slices

Foods in this group include: turkey, fish, chicken, shrimp, crab,
lobster, tofu, egg whites and beans. Red meats may be included,
but should be limited to 2 servings/week.

Dairy

ADULTS AND CHILDREN: 2 - 3 servings/day
ADOLESCENT GIRLS AND WOMEN: 3 - 4 servings/day

SERVING SIZE
milk, yogurt or cottage cheese = 1 cup
hard cheese = 1¹/2 ounces
processed cheese = 1 slice

Note: dairy should be restricted to either skim or low-fat milk
and low-fat milk products.

chapter seven

Getting Started

Getting started is very easy because the Next Generation Fitness plan is quite intuitive once you understand the importance of good nutrition and the basic food color categories. It is designed to accommodate all different tastes and cuisines and to help ensure that you eat colorful, healthy foods every day.

Look at the food chart and color categories on the following pages and pick out foods from each color category that you know you and your family will eat. Note that the list does not include every food in the color category, but all of the foods here are very nutrient-dense. You can easily add other nutrient-dense foods to the list. Just add them to the corresponding color/food group category. Remember that any additions must be HEALTHY foods. Seaweed, for instance could be added to the green category. Note that there are some foods that do not visually match their color in the category. For example, the white category does not represent white foods, but foods that are all high in protein or dairy foods.

One of the purposes of the color scheme is to make sure that your diet contains a proper balance of vitamins, minerals and phytonutrients. It is also an easy way to keep track of your nutrition for the day. Each color category provides a recommended daily amount for both adults and children over the age of 3.

Remember, children over the age of 2 should also be eating a variety of fruits, vegetables, legumes, proteins and milk products on a daily basis, though in smaller portions. For children from 3-5 years old, start with 1 cup of fruit, 1 cup of vegetables and 3-4 grain servings. Increase these quantities to 1¹/₂-2 cups of both fruits and vegetables and 4-6 grain servings for children from the age of 6 until puberty. From the beginning of puberty, a ***minimum*** of 1¹/₂ cups of fruits, 2 cups of vegetables and 6 servings of grains should be consumed daily. Note that the age at which children start puberty varies, as will their calorie demands; make adjustments as children grow. Once your child has finished puberty, the required amounts will vary from 2-3 cups of fruit, 2¹/₂-4 cups of vegetables and 6-8 grain servings per day.

Obviously there is a range for everyone. The serving sizes for fruits and vegetables can always be increased for larger and more active individuals. The grain servings should generally not exceed 11 per day since this much grain would supply most of the day's calories in the form of carbohydrates; the body needs more variety to satisfy nutritional requirements. Although there are super athletes who may require more food because of their enormous energy output, most people will be quite satisfied with these quantities.

Guidelines

1
Never skip a meal.
Skipping meals will cause your metabolic rate to slow down and will most likely cause you to overcompensate by eating empty calories. You will also miss important nutrients in the day.

2
Plan your meals.
By planning your meals, you can keep track of what you are eating so you are more likely to include all the food categories. Without planning, you may find yourself in a situation in which

you are very hungry with no easily available healthy food choices and it is at these times that the temptation to eat junk foods and empty calories will be harder to resist.

3
Fulfill the fruit, vegetable, protein, grain, nuts & dairy requirements each day.
This will keep your from being hungry and you will be less likely to look for empty calorie foods.

4
Avoid deep fried foods.
Have foods that have been sautéed, baked, broiled, roasted, boiled or grilled, NOT deep fried.

5
Exercise.
Do the exercises on the DVD at least three days a week. Physical activity is critical to a healthy future. The current recommended amount of exercise is 30-60 minutes a day, on most days of the week. But the 60 minutes does not have to be done all at once. Breaking it up into 10-15 minute clips makes this goal easily achievable.

6
Involve the entire family.
The whole family's involvement will ensure that this program is a success.

7
No preserved meats!
Most preserved meats contain nitrites which are converted in our bodies to a carcinogen (cancer-causing agent). This includes foods like bologna, salami, pepperoni, hot dogs, corned beef and pastrami.

8

No sodas, juice drinks or sweetened drinks.

Drink mostly water, but include skim or low-fat milk, 100% fruit juices and fresh vegetable juices. Fresh brewed teas, like green teas, can and should be included. Just a reminder: many teas contain caffeine and may have unwanted stimulatory effects on younger children.

GREEN	RED	ORANGE	WHITE
1 CUP	1 CUP	1 CUP	Daily Requirement 2 Protein & 2-3 Dairy Servings*
spinach	tomatoes	butternut squash	turkey
broccoli	tomato sauce	carrots	fish, shrimp crab, lobster & fatty fish
bok choy	red peppers	orange peppers	chicken
peas	apples (any color)	sweet potatoes	egg whites
avocados	cherries	cantaloupe	beans (lentils, chick peas, kidney beans, etc.)
green beans	grapefruit	mango	lean meats
kiwi	strawberries	oranges	nonfat or low-fat dairy products
brussels sprouts	raspberries	papaya	
olives (½ cup limit)	watermelon	pumpkin	

*Serving size for proteins should be approximately the size of a deck of cards; serving size for dairy should be 1 cup skim milk, yogurt or cottage cheese, 1½ ounces hard cheese, or 1 slice of processed cheese.

B	**B**	**Y**	**G**

BLUE	BROWN	YELLOW	GREEN
½ CUP	Daily Requirement 6-11 Grain & 1 Nut Serving*	1 CUP	½ CUP
eggplant	*nuts: 1-2 tbsp.	bananas	dark green leafy lettuce
blackberries	whole wheat pasta	corn (actually a grain)	artichokes
blueberries	whole oats	yellow peppers	kale
grapes	bulgar	pineapple	asparagus
plums	whole grain breads	peaches	soybeans
	whole grain cereals	pears	sea vegetables
	brown rice		honeydew
	wheat germ		
	air-popped popcorn		
	barley		
	buckwheat		
	wild rice		
	whole wheat quinoa		

*1 serving equals 2 tablespoons of nuts

Grow BYG with Color

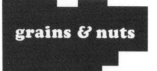

BROWN

Grains

Start your daily planning process with the **BROWN** category, which includes nuts and grains. Grains supply your body with carbohydrates as well as many micronutrients. The body breaks down carbohydrates into glucose. Almost all the reactions that occur in our body require energy supplied by glucose. Also note that whole grains are best and should be included in the diet as often as possible. The most nutritious portion of the grain is stripped off in the refining process, losing a good portion of the phytonutrients. This makes food products with refined carbohydrates a much less nutritionally dense choice. When transitioning to a healthy nutrition plan, you can introduce the whole grains slowly over a period of a few months.

Although many weight-loss programs promote a low-carbohydrate diet, carbohydrates are needed for growth, energy and development and are especially important for children in their growing years. Removing carbohydrates from a child's diet over prolonged periods of time could potentially stunt growth. Low-carbohydrate nutrition plans are NOT healthy diets for anyone.

Nuts

The **BROWN** category also includes nuts. Nuts are a nutritious addition to any meal plan. They contain unsaturated fats, vitamins and minerals and they do not contain cholesterol. Have 2 tablespoons each day, and mix up the variety because they all offer something special. But remember to eat a MAXIMUM of 2 tablespoons per day because they do contain lots of calories. Use caution with young children when first introducing nuts. Allergies to these foods are very serious and can be life-threatening.

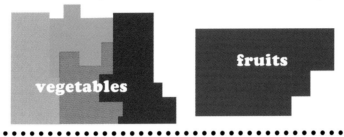

GREEN, ORANGE, RED, BLUE & YELLOW

Fruits

Consuming fruits from all of the different color categories will ensure that your body receives many different vitamins, minerals and phytonutrients. The benefits of eating fruits on a daily basis are well-known. They offer a plethora of nutrients, some of which are still being discovered.[1] Mix up the colors and you'll be sure to meet the nutritional needs of your family.

Vegetables

Vegetables are very important because of their nutritional value as well as their relatively low caloric value, i.e., they are nutritionally dense foods. The red, green, orange, yellow and blue categories have many vegetable choices that all offer different types of nutrients. Feel free to add vegetables to a color category, but try to make sure they are nutrient-dense choices. For example, cucumbers are not listed on the food chart because they are not a nutrient-dense food; though low in calories, cucumbers are not packed with nutrients. This does not preclude eating cucumbers but for the children who have small appetites it is prudent to fill them with a more nutrient-dense food. Cucumbers can be a great addition for people with larger appetites who tend to overeat.

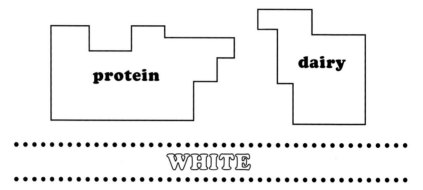

WHITE

Proteins

Proteins are the building blocks for muscles, enzymes and cells. Notice that not every food in the white category is actually white; however, the foods in this category are all high in protein. Each food on the chart is nutrient-rich and low in saturated fat. You may also have noticed that there is no beef, veal, pork or lamb included in the plan. You can eat these meats, but limit them to once or twice per week because they are higher in saturated fat than poultry and fish.

Dairy

The **WHITE** category also includes all dairy products. Dairy products provide calcium, the main structural component of our bones. If children do not get enough calcium, along with exercise, their future bone health is at risk.

So Where's the Fat?

You may have observed that fat is not included in any of the categories; nor is there a separate fat category. However, this does not mean that there is no fat in this nutrition plan. Fats are the molecules that give cells structure, protect our organs and protect us during periods of illness and any prolonged decrease in calorie intake. Fats are important substances and they are needed to maintain a healthy body. Everyone over the age of 2 should have 20-30 percent of their caloric intake from fat. Children under the age of 2 require even more fat (up to 50 percent of their calories) in their diet for brain growth. Breast milk should be the main source of fat for brain growth in the first year of life. During the second year of life, babies will transition to whole cow's milk which supplies the main source of fat for the toddler. It is hard to avoid fat so don't worry that you might get too little. Only a very disciplined person will be able to restrict fat intake to less than 20 percent of daily calories.

Most people get sufficient fats from the foods included in this nutritional plan. Using only 1-2 tablespoons of ***added*** fat per day, for example, fats that you add to food like salad dressing, is enough for most people. The more common problem is making sure that you are not consuming too much fat. Many food packages now list the percent of calories in the food that come from fat. Avoid foods that have a total of more than 30 percent of their caloric value in fat.

When cooking, use oil that is made mainly from polyunsaturated or monounsaturated fats like olive oil or canola oil. Eat avocados, soybeans, nuts and olives. The fats in these foods tend to lower cholesterol levels and can decrease risk for heart disease. Other good sources of these fats are fatty fish like salmon, herring, mackerel and tuna. The fats in these fish contain omega-3 fatty acids that are easily converted to anti-inflammatory and anti-clotting agents. Other foods that contain omega-3 fatty acids are walnuts, flax meal and some plant foods. We should consume a variety of foods that contain omega-3 fatty acids on a regular basis.

Saturated fats are found in animal products, dairy products and some vegetable oils. Animal products also contain cholesterol. Although our body naturally manufactures cholesterol, eating these foods increases cholesterol levels. Elevated cholesterol levels are related to an increased risk of heart disease. We should limit our intake of saturated fats and cholesterol-laden foods.

Mix It Up

The Next Generation Fitness plan is very flexible, making it easier to be successful. There are many foods to choose from and enough to keep you from ever being hungry. You may have more than one serving of a food in each category, but try to mix it up as best as you can to include all the categories. If you pick a high carbohydrate vegetable from one category, try to pick a low carbohydrate choice from another color category. Use lots of onions and garlic while cooking; they are loaded with disease-preventing phytonutrients.

Most people tend to eat the same meals over and over again, though perhaps prepared somewhat differently for variety. If each of our meals consists only of two or three different types of foods, this usually gives us nine different food options to rotate throughout the day. If we are choosing from among the same foods for our meals, very little thought will be needed to plan most of our basic meals. This makes it easy to plan and to keep track of what you are eating. It is important to keep track of the amount of all the foods that you eat on a daily basis, especially in the beginning when it is not yet a habit.

When I consult with families about diet and nutrition, I suggest two or three main meal choices for breakfast, lunch and dinner, making sure that colorful fruits and vegetables are used as well as lean meats, fish or beans and whole grains. This type of planning makes it easy to ensure that you include a wide variety of vegetables, fruits, protein and grains each day. The easier things are, the more likely you will be to follow through with plans and be successful.

Start setting your goals and look forward to a healthier future!

chapter eight

Planning a Nutritious Day

This is an easy-to-follow, step-by-step example of how to plan a nutrient-filled day for you and your children. This sample illustrates how to build a daily nutrition plan for one adult. Use it as a model for making your own personalized plan using the template on page 214. For each step, fill in your choice of foods from each category. Use the portion guidelines shown on pages 68-70 to determine the quantities and adjust the portion sizes for children. When you have completed the chart, you will have your own plan for the day. Select a variety of foods for other days—you'll find that it gets even easier as you use it more frequently and as you get more familiar with what foods are in each category. Healthy eating!

1

Plan your grains and nuts for the day.

(See BROWN category, page 68.)

Note that each of the grain portions contains 2
serving sizes, giving you a total of 6 portions.
Six servings of grains is a good place for most adults to start.

STEP 1: Starting with GRAINS & NUTS	Portion Size
Breakfast	oatmeal	1 cup
Snack	nuts	2 tbsp. (maximum)
Lunch	whole wheat bread for sandwich	2 slices
Snack		
Dinner	pasta	1 cup
Snack		

2

Now add fruit to your daily meal plan.

*(See GREEN, ORANGE, RED, BLUE & YELLOW category,
page 69.)*

By adding 3 fruits, you have satisfied
your fruit requirements for the day.

STEP 2: Adding FRUITS to the plan	Portion Size
Breakfast	oatmeal	1 cup
	blueberries	1/2 cup
Snack	nuts	2 tablespoons
Lunch	whole wheat bread (for sandwich)	2 slices
Snack	orange	1 medium-sized
Dinner	pasta	1 cup
Snack	strawberries	1/2 cup

3
Next add vegetables to the plan to meet the daily requirements.

(See GREEN, ORANGE, RED, BLUE & YELLOW category, page 69.)

STEP 3: Adding VEGETABLES to the plan	Portion Size
Breakfast oatmeal	1 cup
blueberries	1/2 cup
Snack nuts	2 tablespoons
Lunch whole wheat bread (for sandwich)	2 slices
leafy vegetables	**1 cup**
tomatoes	**1/2 cup**
Snack orange	1 medium-sized
Dinner pasta	1 cup
broccoli	**1 1/2 cups**
Snack strawberries	1/2 cup

4
Continue by adding dairy products to your plan.
Remember that adolescent and adult females
need 3-4 dairy servings per day,
while younger children and adults need 2-3 servings.
(See WHITE category, page 70.)

STEP 4: Adding DAIRY to the plan		Portion Size
Breakfast	oatmeal	1 cup
	blueberries	1/2 cup
	skim milk	**1 cup**
Snack	nuts	2 tablespoons
Lunch	whole wheat bread (for sandwich)	2 slices
	leafy vegetables	1 cup
	tomatoes	1/2 cup
Snack	orange	1 medium-sized
Dinner	pasta	1 cup
	broccoli	1 1/2 cups
Snack	strawberries	1/2 cup
	low-fat or nonfat yogurt	**1 cup**

5
Now add the protein.
(See WHITE category, page 70.)

STEP 5: Adding PROTEIN to the plan		Portion Size	Color Group Servings
Breakfast	oatmeal	1 cup	2 Brown
	blueberries	1/2 cup	1/2 Blue
	skim milk	1 cup	1 White Dairy
Snack	nuts	2 tablespoons	1 Brown
Lunch	whole wheat bread (for sandwich)	2 slices	2 Brown
	turkey slices	**3 slices**	**1 White Protein**
	leafy vegetables	1 cup	1/2 Green
	tomatoes	1/2 cup	1/2 Red
Snack	orange	1 medium-sized	1 Orange
Dinner	pasta	1 cup	2 Brown
	broccoli	1 1/2 cups	1 1/2 Green
	chicken breast	**4 oz.** (about the size of a deck of cards)	**1 White Protein**
Snack	strawberries	1/2 cup	1/2 Red
	nonfat yogurt	1 cup	1 White Dairy

6
Let's not forget about staying well hydrated.

The best drink to have is water. Skim milk and
100 percent fruit juices are also good ways to incorporate
nutrients with fluid into the diet. Children need at least
6 glasses of fluids a day; adults need to have 8 glasses per day.

Just remember the colors by saying:

GROW BYG

G = GREEN

R = RED

O = ORANGE

W = WHITE

B = BLUE, BROWN

Y = YELLOW

See APPENDIX 4, for a handy nutrition guide; APPENDIX 5, for a blank chart you can copy and use for your daily planning and APPENDIX 6, for a quick reference chart of portion sizes.

The chart on page 89 shows samples of some typical meals or snacks and how the ingredients in these menu items satisfy both the color categories and serving portions of the daily requirement of the plan. You can see how colorful meals can be appealing and healthy. When putting together meals and menus, you can combine groups and colors. Not only will your meal be more colorful, you will easily satisfy several of your daily requirements.

FOOD	Green	Red	Orange	White	Blue	Brown	Yellow	Added Advantages
1 cup of low-fat yogurt with 1/2 cup of blueberries, 1 tbsp. wheat germ & 2 tbsp. of nuts				1 milk serving	1/2 cup	1 nut serving		packed with vitamins & phyto-nutrients
1 cup oatmeal with banana						2 servings	1 cup	
1 small whole wheat baked tortilla with 1 cup spinach dip	1 cup			1/2 milk serving		1 serving		lots of nutrients, vitamins, & minerals
3 oz. chicken breast with peppers on small whole wheat bun		1/2 cup		1 protein serving		2 servings		
2 cups chopped salad with 1/2 cup tomatoes, 1/2 orange, 1/2 cup orange peppers and 1 cup shrimp & beans	1 cup	1/2 cup	1 cup	1 serving protein (beans & shrimp)				
2 tbsp. peanut butter & jelly on whole wheat bread		1/4 cup				1 nut serving 2 brown servings		only use jelly with no added sugar
bagel (average size bagel) with 2 thin slices of low-fat cheese				1 milk serving		4 servings		whole wheat bagel adds more fiber

Keep It Fun
For the Whole Family

Once you get started, you will find that you and your family can have fun with the Next Generation Fitness Program. By keeping track of the colors of the foods you eat each day, you are less likely to miss a major food category and you will get a variety of nutrients. Also, even young children can follow and understand color categories. Anything that makes it easier for children will ultimately make it easier for the parents. Ideally, this program should begin as soon as children are ready to eat solid foods (about 9 months for most children). Getting kids used to eating vegetables, fruits and legumes when they are very young will make it that much easier as they grow. And it will probably avoid conflicts later on about the chicken nugget and French fry diet. Even if your children are older, however, it's not too late to start. Enlist them in sorting their daily meals into color categories and be creative in inventing games so they can participate in the planning.

Because most people eat the same types of foods on a rotating basis, it becomes very easy to make sure that we include most food colors in our daily plan. As you plan your food for the day, just think of the colors and adjust your choice of fruit of vegetables to meet your nutrition needs. If children are raised with the concept of eating a colorful diet, it will become a habit that is naturally followed into adulthood. The Next Generation Fitness Program will give your children a better chance at a healthier future.

Why Are Colors Important?

We know that eating fruits and vegetables on a regular basis will create a healthy body and the antioxidants in these foods contribute to this. But we also need to understand why the food color categories are so important. The pigments that give foods their color contain most of the phytonutrients that protect our health. Different color pigments contain different nutrients; it is essential to get a variety of colors in our daily diet in order to get all the needed nutrients for optimum health.

Following is a list of the food colors and what makes them special. This list is not all-inclusive; research continues to discover more and more reasons for us to consume these colorful foods. Not every food in its color category provides all the benefits listed and some foods have benefits that are not listed. The following are just some of the reasons that children need to get in the habit of eating some foods from each group on a daily basis.

GREEN FRUITS & VEGETABLES

* Vitamin K to heal wounds
* Lutein and zeaxanthin to protect against cataracts
* Bioflavonoids and Vitamin C for immune system and skin health
* Potassium, calcium and magnesium for blood pressure
* Isothiocynates to deactivate cancer-causing agents
* Plant sterols to decrease cholesterol absorption
* Isoflavones to increase "good" cholesterol

RED FRUITS & VEGETABLES

* Lycopene and monoterpenes for cancer and heart protection
* Vitamin C for immune system, skin and blood vessels
* Soluble fiber to decrease "bad" cholesterol
* Antioxidants to protect cells from damage that leads to heart disease, cancer, stroke, dementia, etc.

ORANGE FRUITS & VEGETABLES

* Alpha and beta carotene as antioxidants to protect the cells and the skin from sun damage

* Vitamin C as an antioxidant to protect bones, skin, blood vessels and the immune system

* Folic acid to prevent neural tube defects in the developing fetus

* Naringin to protect against heart disease, cancer, improve bone formation and glucose utilization

WHITE CATEGORY: PROTEIN & DAIRY

* Protein for essential body functions: maintaining and building muscle, creating enzymes for our body to use energy, building new cells and fighting off infection

* Calcium and vitamin D to manufacture strong bones and teeth (DAIRY ONLY)

* Zinc for use in over 100 enzymes needed for the body to function

* Iron for healthy blood

* Selenium for the body's natural antioxidant system

BLUE FRUITS & VEGETABLES

* Antioxidants to protect against heart disease, cancer and stroke

* Fiber to decrease cholesterol

* Vitamin C for the immune system and skin health

YELLOW FRUITS & VEGETABLES

* Potassium and magnesium to maintain a healthy blood pressure

* Vitamin B_6 for use in protein metabolism and to maintain a healthy nervous system

BROWN CATEGORY: WHOLE GRAINS & NUTS

GRAINS

* B vitamins to metabolize our food and convert it to energy

* Fiber for a healthy colon

* Thiamin for use in nerves and muscle function

* Zinc for use in every cell in the body

* Iron needed for transport of oxygen to the cells in the body

NUTS
(Very important, and often overlooked)

* Vitamin E, a potent antioxidant

* Omega-3 fatty acids as an anti-inflammatory and for heart health

* Copper for proper functioning of enzymes

Frequently Asked Questions:

Nutrition

1
Q) Does fast food fit in to this plan?

A) No, but this does not mean that your child cannot ever have these foods. You need to recognize that these items should only be eaten sparingly. Nutrient-deficient foods do more harm than good. Try to offer healthier substitutions instead, e.g., baked chicken versus chicken nuggets, frozen yogurt versus ice cream.

When these foods are eaten on occasion, it is recommended that you adjust the overall intake for the day. For example if your child eats cake at a birthday party, swap it out for one grain serving and try not to choose additional high-fat foods for that day.

2
Q) Can I have pizza?

A) Yes, but try to have pizza without the cheese. Instead, have salad, bruschetta or vegetable slices. One average slice with cheese can be broken down as 3 BROWN (grain) servings, 2 WHITE (dairy) servings and 1/2 RED (vegetable) serving. The cheese on regular pizza is high-fat cheese, so limit this choice.

3
Q) Can we drink flavored waters? And what about sports drinks?

A) It is very important that everyone consume enough fluids to keep hydrated. Plain water is the healthiest choice; however, flavored varieties are acceptable. If your children prefer these, it might be helpful to try to use fresh lemons and limes to make your own, without any artificial sweeteners. Sugary sport drinks are similar to sodas and fruit drinks in that they contain more sugar than the body needs. It is recommended that you remove these types of drinks from the diet.

4
Q) Isn't it true that nuts are bad for you because they are fattening?

A) No. There is a major misconception about the nutrition of nuts. Nuts are high in fat; however, these are "good" (i.e., unsaturated) fats. Nuts also contain essential vitamins and minerals that are beneficial to our bodies, are a great source of protein and have actually been shown to ward off hunger considerably longer than other foods that are high in fat.[1] Nuts are high in calories so you need to control your portions. But they should be incorporated into your meal plan. The best nuts to choose are almonds, cashews, walnuts and peanuts. If you or your family have nut allergies, it would be beneficial to try to incorporate flax meal or wheat germ instead, as they provide similar nutritional benefits.

5
Q) Do I have to eat every color food each day?

A) No. Try to have as many colors as you can each day. You will get used to thinking about the colors of the foods that you like to eat. The more variety, the better balance you will have internally.

6
Q) Can I add other foods to the list?

A) Yes, but these foods should be healthy, nutrient-filled items. For example, you may be a pickle lover. Although pickles are a vegetable, they have little nutrient value, and pickling adds way too much salt. If you like cucumbers, you can certainly eat them, but remember that they are not very nutritious.

7

Q) Is it necessary to take vitamins if I am following this nutrition plan?

A) Menstruating females need to take a vitamin supplement to supply them with enough iron. Adult men who are eating a balanced diet full of vegetables, fruits and whole grains do not need vitamin supplements. Children who eat a well-balanced diet also do not need additional vitamins. Unfortunately, this is all too rare and most children will need supplements. In areas where there is no fluoride in the water, a pediatrician will give prescription vitamins to supply fluoride.

8

Q) What if my child eats only one or two colors of fruits and vegetables?

A) If your child will only eat broccoli and red peppers and refuses to eat any of the foods in other color groups, follow the steps on page 28 and continually introduce new foods.

9

Q) Are there any foods that the family can eat in unlimited quantity?

A) Next Generation Fitness includes a nutrition plan that teaches the principles of a balanced diet and portion control. There are "diet plans" that make recommendations on foods that can be eaten in unlimited quantities. These foods are usually devoid of nutrition and mainly consist of water. If hunger is an issue when trying to follow a healthy lifestyle, fill yourself up with water before meals, eat very slowly and take breaks while eating.

10

Q) Is it safe to give children artificial sweeteners like aspartame?

A) The artificial sweeteners on the market are generally regarded as safe and can be used by everyone. However, knowing that they are safe does not give a green light to ingesting large quantities of them. Limit their use and drink mostly water, skim milk, 100 percent fruit juices, vegetable juices and green tea.

11

Q) Apples come in different colors. If I eat a green apple should I put it in the green category?

A) There are a wide variety of apples. For simplicity sake, all apples regardless of color should be classified in the red category.

12

Q) Is it okay to give my child decaffeinated teas?

A) Using decaffeinated products is perfectly acceptable. Since most of the tea antioxidants are heat stable, there should be plenty of health benefits to the decaffeinated versions.

chapter nine

The Exercise Program

One of the three variables that I evaluate during a child's check-up is how much exercise the child is getting. This issue presents a big challenge. Time for exercise competes directly with computers, videogames, cell phones and television, all of which are sedentary activities that children generally find more entertaining than exercise. In prior generations, if a child wanted to play with friends, the child walked to the friend's home and the children played outside. In today's world, children interact through online games and text messaging, and they play mesmerizing home videogames that are often solitary activities. Parents must set limits on these nonproductive, sedentary activities. When limits are not set, children will continue these activities indefinitely. These are passive activities and it is always easier to choose the path of least resistance. It is up to parents to intervene and make changes; children will never opt to end these activities on their own. Our children are so dependent on being entertained all the time that some manufacturers have built in videos to their exercise equipment so that children can be entertained while they work out.

Studies have made it quite clear that regular exercising is likely to increase our life span because of the beneficial effects of exercise on heart muscles, bones, mental acuity, mood and blood pressure. In addition, exercising can even help prevent diseases like osteoporosis, type II diabetes, colon cancer and heart disease.[1] In spite of this knowledge, most people—adults as well as children—do not get the recommended amount of exercise each day. The goal of the Next Generation Fitness Program is to exercise 6 days a week for 30-60 minutes each day. This may seem like a lot and therefore feels unattainable, but it is easier than you think. The exercise does not have to be done all at once. It is perfectly okay to do 5-10 minutes at a time.

A typical day for a child should involve lots of running around and playing games outdoors. This activity of course counts as exercise. However, even those children who are physically active need to acquire the *exercise habit*. This is a new concept for children as well as adults, but it is an essential one. In order for children to form this habit, we need to teach them how to exercise at home, without fancy equipment.

The Next Generation Fitness DVD can help us achieve this goal. The DVD shows children how to do simple exercises. Once learned, these exercises can be continued into adulthood. They can be done anywhere and ideally, parents should exercise along with their children. This reinforces the habit, provides a regular family activity and keeps the whole family healthier.

The DVD contains three separate workouts that offer resistance training combined with aerobic exercise. Resistance training uses a weight that acts as resistance to build muscle. It is not recommended that children use dumbbells or go to unsupervised gyms that are not approved for child use for this kind of exercise. The exercises in the Next Generation Fitness Program teach children to use their body weight as the resistance. Doing push-ups, pull-ups, sit-ups, chin-ups, squats or tricep dips is a great way to resistance train. There is nothing better or more convenient than pulling your own body weight as a form of resistance training.

Exercise is the most neglected aspect of children's health and therefore it is the one that requires the most focus. Although our lives are busy, they are frequently sedentary; when we do have free time, exercise is not usually our first choice for an activity. We need to get motivated in order to motivate our children. The parents of children who play team sports and participate on two or three teams during the year are often fooled into thinking that their child is getting sufficient exercise. This is false. Children need to be taught how to exercise without a team and they must get into the habit of exercising at home so that it becomes part of their daily routine. Use the DVD to teach your children how to exercise without a team, reinforce the importance of resistance training, encourage daily home exercise and be a good role model.

Resistance Training

This is a crucial part of any exercise program, but most exercise programs for children do not include resistance training. The Next Generation Fitness workout program uses the body's own weight as the resistance, and it is the safest way for children and adolescents to weight train without using dumbbells. Resistance training helps to increase strength, improve bone formation, increase muscle mass and increase metabolic rate.[2] The increase in muscle mass is very important; when a decrease in energy intake occurs during dieting or illness, our muscles serve as a reservoir to maintain blood sugar. Resistance training does not build muscle in prepubertal children, but it WILL increase strength, balance, stamina and bone density.[3] Increasing bone density when you are young is crucial in helping to stave off osteoporosis and possible bone fractures as you age. Resistance training needs to be a part of all exercise programs, including those for children.

Aerobic Exercise

This part of the workout exercises the heart. The benefits of cardiac exercise are well known: It helps with heart health and blood pressure, increases the "good" cholesterol and helps to maintain a healthy body weight.

Increased Energy Habits

The list below provides some suggestions for ways your family can exercise together. It also offers some ideas about how you can increase your energy expenditure and burn more calories each day. Some of these are simple and will easily fit into your daily routine. Others may require some planning. Try to incorporate a few of these activities into your exercise routines every day. These additional boosters are not replacements for the exercises on the DVD; rather, they are ways to make some of your daily activities more active and get more exercise from things you are already doing. Take into account the time you spend on these activities; if done vigorously, count them as part of the time you spend on your daily exercise.

WALK instead of getting in the car. Involve the whole family in fun walks in parks, around the block, to the grocery store, etc. (Parents should always accompany children, as appropriate for age and location.) A brisk pace when walking is better than a leisurely pace. Using a pedometer is lots of fun for kids; they enjoy keeping track of how far they walk in a day. Sometimes it is quite surprising to see how much (or little) walking is done doing daily activities. I wore a pedometer in my office for a few weeks and discovered, to my surprise, that I had walked an average of three miles each day in the office! When shopping, find a parking spot farther away from the store. The longer walk will increase your heart rate and if you are carrying packages, you'll get the added benefit of a resistance workout!

STAIR CLIMBING is a wonderful addition to the day. If your home has stairs, use them even when you don't have to, and get your heart rate up and work your leg muscles. If you live in a building that has an elevator (or work in one or visit such buildings on a regular basis), use the stairs instead of the elevator whenever possible (within a reasonable number of flights of stairs). Remember to use the stairs whenever you can. They can provide a quick aerobic activity that takes only a few extra minutes.

BIKE RIDING is always a fun activity and it can be enjoyed by the whole family. Encourage family outings on bike trails. Bicycle riding is a great cardiovascular activity and it also provides some resistance training to the lower body. Remember: Everyone should always wear a bicycle helmet.

PLAY OUTDOOR GAMES such as catch, tag, hopscotch, hide and seek, etc. Childhood games can be great family fun, regardless of age.

SWIMMING is one of the best exercises but is limited by climate, weather and access. If your children have access to swimming pools, encourage them to make use of the facilities as long as they are supervised. Reinforce the importance of never swimming alone. In the summer most children do not need to be encouraged to play in a swimming pool. For those children who would rather play videogames, parents should encourage swimming; it is a source of fun as well as excellent physical exercise because it exercises every muscle in your body. If your child feels uncomfortable in a bathing suit, supplying a T-shirt as a cover-up usually helps.

HOUSEHOLD CHORES can be an excellent source of exercise. Everyday activities like carrying groceries, taking out the garbage, vacuuming, dusting and washing clothes will provide some calorie-burning activity and help develop a sense of responsibility. Get your children to share in these chores if they don't already do so, but turn them into fun exercise moments instead of chores. Chores can be fun and give a child a sense of accomplishment. Play music and dance around while vacuuming, or see who can carry in the groceries the fastest. Make games out of chores and they won't be "chores" but instead ways to work your body, have fun and give you a feeling of accomplishment.

SHOVELING SNOW when the weather has provided the right conditions is excellent aerobic exercise. Clearing snow from driveways and walkways is a very vigorous physical activity. It will help build upper and lower body strength and give you a cardiac workout. When lifting, you have to bend the knees and let your legs help lift the load to protect your back. Shoveling snow will also give you a resistance workout. But remember, everyone needs to be careful not to overdo it. A caution to adults: shoveling snow can be a ***very vigorous workout***; for those who are not in shape it can be harmful and even dangerous.

GARDENING can be a wonderful way to keep active as well as keep the outside of your house looking beautiful. Children love seeing their efforts grow into flowers and many children enjoy the rewards of a vegetable garden. Planting, weeding and picking flowers and/or fruits and vegetables can be a good source of exercise that also provides a sense of accomplishment. Some of the rewards may even be incorporated into your meal plans!

The Home Workout

The Next Generation Fitness workout program is designed for use at home. The only equipment recommended is a pull-up bar and a large exercise ball, but the DVD can be used without them. The DVD contains three 20-30-minute workout programs. Each program contains workout sets broken into 1-2 minutes of alternating resistance exercises and cardiac exercises. The child's weight is used to resistance train with basic exercises like sit-ups, push-ups, squat thrusts, tricep dips and pull-ups. The cardiac exercises are simple exercises like jumping jacks and running in place and are very easy for any child to do. The exercises demonstrated in each program will work most major muscles in the body. As your level of fitness improves, you can increase the number of times you repeat each exercise in each set. *The goal is to continually increase the repetitions in each set.*

Stretching is also an important part of any workout. The stretches are introduced at the beginning of each of the DVD programs. Stretches are then included again at the end of each program. It is important to maximize the stretching to ensure that you keep limber. Stretching is a commonly overlooked area of children's sports. Many preteen sports practices involve **just** performing sport-specific skills. Many coaches of these teams are generous and involved parents who donate their time, and they do a great job, but they are not trainers or physical education teachers. Children must learn how to stay limber; being limber will help to decrease the risk of sports-related injuries. I have observed over the many years in pediatric practice that children's weakest area often involves the hamstring muscles. So many of my young athletes have such tight hamstring muscles that it is hard for them to bend forward during a scoliosis check. Tight hamstring muscles can lead to chronic lower back pain in adulthood. I tell every patient who has tight hamstrings to do stretching exercises routinely, and I explain why stretching is important for everyone. Tightness of these muscles in adults can also lead to chronic back pain. Adequate stretching is important for everyone who wants a healthier body.

The Next Generation Fitness workout is challenging! If at first you can't do the recommended number of exercises per set, decrease the number of repetitions but try to do at least one or two in each set. The more frequently you use the program, the stronger you will become. You will also receive the added benefit of increasing your metabolic rate. Your metabolic rate increases during any physical activity and even after the activity. The time that it takes for your metabolic rate to slow to resting depends on the duration and intensity of the exercise. During strenuous and prolonged physical activity, the metabolic rate remains elevated for about two hours, but more importantly, as you increase muscle mass and muscle usage, your resting metabolic rate (not to be confused with heart rate) will increase permanently over time. This will help with maintaining a healthy weight or losing weight for those who need it. Remember to alternate Exercise Programs 1, 2 and 3 on different days of the week. You should not do the same resistance exercises on consecutive days. This will allow your muscles to recover.

HYDRATION IS IMPORTANT. Drink water before beginning the exercises, and then continue to drink in between exercises and at the end of the workout. The recommended amount of water is 4-6 ounces for younger children per 20-30 minutes of exercise, and 8-12 ounces of water for adolescents/adults per 20-30 minutes of exercise.[4]

It is important to pay attention to proper form and good posture while exercising. While doing any standing exercises, make sure that your shoulders are back and your spine is straight. NO SLOUCHING! Viewing yourself in a mirror while you exercise will help to ensure good form. You will always get more out of a workout if you perform the stretches and exercises correctly and more importantly, if you don't perform the exercises correctly, you may increase the risk for injury. *You should never feel pain while working out.* It is normal to feel a slight aching sensation while working out, but it is never normal to feel sharp, tingling or cramping pain. These are signals to stop what you are doing, and if the pain persists, get evaluated by your doctor.

Exercising should be fun and stimulating so try to have a good time. To help motivate you, think about the positive aspects of exercising and visualize what you are accomplishing. Most people will start to see a difference in 1-2 weeks of exercising and eating well, but everyone will **feel** the difference immediately. Visualize yourself as stronger and firmer; imagine yourself having more endurance and more energy. Help your children visualize themselves performing better on their sports team, jumping higher or running longer. Having more energy, feeling better and improving school performance are always good motivators. However, we must keep in mind that this program is not about looks or weight: it's about our health. It's critical that children understand this concept and that we do not focus on a child's weight or looks. Children's visualizations must emphasize other aspects of a healthy lifestyle rather than how they will look if they loose weight.

You can also use visualization techniques for other physical activities to help with motivating you and your family. For example, before setting out for a family bike ride, focus on the destination, and those hills along the way may not seem so hard to climb. Form a mental image of firmer, stronger legs. Keep motivated by thinking of the reasons to stay physically fit and each exercise you do will be that much more enjoyable. Visualize stronger legs and a body that is more limber and agile. As you exercise more regularly, your body will be in better condition and will become more flexible, leaving you less susceptible to injury.

Finally, the Next Generation Fitness Program will also increase your stamina because you are exercising the most important muscle of all: your heart!

ENJOY YOUR WORKOUT!!!

Frequently Asked Questions: Exercise

1

Q) Why does my child need to do the workout DVD if she is already playing on sports teams?

A) Parents, do not be fooled! Your child may be involved in three or four different sports and you may therefore feel he/she does not need an exercise program. This is a big mistake. Children need to learn HOW to exercise apart from their sports team. You need to get children into the HABIT of an exercise routine that they can use both while they are part of a sports team AND after the sport season is over! Resistance training is generally not included as part of any sports team training in schools but the benefits of the use of *proper resistance training* in children cannot be overemphasized! I used the words "proper resistance training" because there is a correct form to working out a particular muscle group; if lifting weights is not done properly, children are open to injury. It is also important to know how to choose the correct weight to lift; most boys will try to lift as much weight as they are able. This is called a maximal lift and can cause muscle, ligament or tendon damage.

2

Q) What if we cannot do all the segments on the DVD?

A) Do as many segments as you can. Many people cannot do all the exercises the first time they go through the program. It may take time before you can accomplish this. Try to do as many as you can. If you feel you cannot hold on to the bar any longer, it is time to let go and take a rest. Keep track of how many repetitions you do, and try to increase them by one or two each time you do the exercise. Your strength and fitness level will improve as long as you continue with the program!

3

Q) Isn't gym class in school enough exercise?

A) No! Most schools do not give children exercises that they can continue to do at home and time is very limited in school. Gym classes are very important because they give children a chance to exercise during the day and play sports with their classmates. Most gym classes include some kind of aerobics, whether as exercises or as part of a sport during the class. But gym classes rarely involve resistance training, even though this is as important as the aerobics.

4

Q) Will my child develop big muscles if he does this workout?

A) Prepubertal children do not significantly increase muscle size through resistance training. They will, however, increase strength and bone density and improve their ability to use their muscles. Boys who are going through puberty or have gone through puberty will increase muscle size naturally. The degree of this increase depends on what they are eating, genetics and how much resistance training they do. Girls who are going through or have gone through puberty can also increase their muscle size and strength, but to a much lesser extent than boys.

5

Q) What if my child complains that he is sore the next day?

A) This is a normal response when formerly unused muscles are suddenly used! Being sore means the muscles have had a good workout. But if you are sore, wait until your muscles feel better before doing exercises that involve these muscles. You can still do other exercises that involve other muscle groups.

6

Q) What if my child complains of pain while working out?

A) Any complaint of pain while working out must be taken seriously! When working our muscles, there are occasions when a slight straining sensation is felt. This is normal. Should you experience a sharp, shooting, cramping or hot pain, however, stop the exercise program. If the pain persists, take your child to the doctor.

7

Q) Why does my child need to workout if he is already thin?

A) It is very important to have and maintain healthy muscles, including your heart. This applies to children as well as adults. Everyone should do both aerobic and resistance exercises, regardless of weight. Increasing muscle size and strength through regular resistance exercise will help to maintain healthy bones, improve posture, tone and endurance. Regular aerobic exercises are needed to maintain a healthy heart. The Next Generation Fitness Program uses a combination of resistance and aerobic training and is appropriate for people of all ages and all weights.

8

Q) Why is resistance training important and is it dangerous for my child?

A) Resistance training is a crucial part of any effective exercise program. Resistance training helps to increase strength, tone and endurance. It builds muscle that can be used by the body if needed in times of severe stress or illness. It will also help to keep bones strong. Resistance training for children has been endorsed by the American Academy of Pediatrics. However, caution must be used. Children should never go into a gym and use weights. It is much better to use a program that focuses on using the weight of your own body as the resistance, which is the most natural way to increase strength. The Next Generation Fitness Program shows you how to do this effectively.

chapter ten

Looking to the Future

Did you ever wonder why some people can eat French fries and milk shakes and never gain weight, AND they have normal cholesterol, while others struggle with their weight and have high cholesterol even though they watch every ounce of fat in their diet? The answer of course is in our genes. Some people's genes are set up to metabolize fat molecules so that they can maintain normal cholesterol, regardless of diet, while others are not. This is not to say that such people do not need to acquire healthy eating habits; all bad eating habits will eventually cause a problem somewhere down the road.

Is it possible to change your genetic programming by changing the way you eat? Do you think we can select a diet that could successfully reduce the chances of developing certain cancers for people who are predisposed to them? Is it possible to generate someone's genetic profile and use it to create a nutrition plan that would keep that person at optimal health? The answer to these questions is YES![1]

Let me give you an example of a gene-nutrition interaction to illustrate how genes and diet affect us on a molecular level. A disease called phenlyketonuria is genetically transmitted. Babies affected by this disease lack the enzyme needed to metabolize the amino acid phenylalanine. Without this enzyme toxic material builds up inside of the body. These toxic substances can cause mental retardation, seizures and death. If identified in infancy (newborn screenings in all states look for this disease), the condition can be handled simply by restricting the amino acid phenylalanine in the diet by limiting intake of certain proteins. Without the phenylalanine, the body does not build up the toxic substances and the baby will grow into a healthy adult. This is but one of many examples of the how changing nutritional intake can stave off a terrible disease before it does damage. This disease is a *relatively* simple one-gene defect, but chronic diseases, like heart disease, obesity, cancers and diabetes, are not due to "simple" one-gene defects. There are many, many genes as well as many complex gene-nutrition interactions that will play a role in whether or not an individual develops these diseases.

The new fields of nutrigenomics and nutrigenetics study nutrition and gene interaction. What we eat affects our genes (nutrigenomics) and our genes shape the body's response to what we eat (nutrigenetics). The fields of nutrigenetics and nutrigenomics are working toward solving questions about how our genetic code can be used to keep us all healthy. Researchers in these fields are working diligently to identify how genes and nutrient interactions allow one person to stay healthy while another may become obese or develop heart disease. If we can identify the genetic interactions that affect diet and nutrition and can test for them, we can personalize an individual's diet to avoid a problem that would otherwise be present. Every day scientists are coming up with new models that help us understand more about the interrelationship between diet, disease and our genetic code.

The Human Genome project, the complete study of the human genetic code, was released in 2003, making it available to researchers. It will be possible to obtain a unique genetic fingerprint for each individual and use this genetic information to specify a diet that will maximize an individual's health.[2]

Stay tuned for future developments!

Recipes

Following are examples of recipes that meet the requirements of the Next Generation Fitness Program: healthy, tasty, low-fat, nutrient-dense meals that are easy to prepare. For your convenience, color codes are provided so you can see at a glance which recipes contain the ingredients from specific food color groups and you can easily track them. This will help get you to start thinking in terms of food colors while planning and eating your meals.

Each recipe includes an extensive nutrient breakdown unique to this book; you will not find this information on food labels or in most other cookbooks or diet books. The recommended daily allowance (RDA) is the amount of a particular nutrient required to prevent deficiency as determined by the National Academy of Science. These numbers are given as a percentage of the total recommended for one day's intake. Also included are some of the "21st century" nutrients that have been described and are a core part of *Growing Up Healthy*. There is no RDA for the intake of these substances so they are expressed as the actual amount found in the serving of food in each recipe. There are some large variations in amounts of some of these nutrients so do not think they are errors; they are just nutrient-dense foods.

You will note that some recipes call for nonstick spray while others use cooking oils. If you decide to use a little olive oil or canola oil instead of a nonstick spray, bear in mind that the calorie and fat content will change.

Breakfast

Fresh Fruit Salad

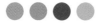

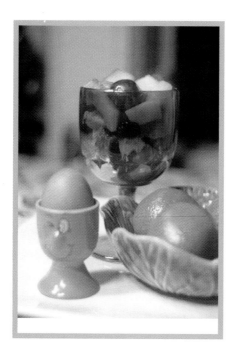

INGREDIENTS

1 cup fresh raspberries

1 cup fresh blueberries

1 cup cantaloupe, cubed

1 cup honeydew, cubed

1 orange, peeled with slices cut into halves

1 tsp. lime zest

2 tbsp. lime juice

PREPARATION

Mix together all ingredients.

Note: *The vitamin C in the lime juice will help keep the fruit from turning color.*

NUTRITION FACTS

Makes 5 servings   Serving size: 1 cup

Total calories per serving	70	Total protein	1g
Total carbohydrates	16g	Total fat	0g
Total fiber	4g	Saturated fat	0g

· ·

% DAILY REQUIREMENT

Vitamin A	24	Vitamin C	69	Vitamin B$_6$	5	Folate	7
Calcium	2	Iron	2	Vitamin B$_{12}$	0	Biotin	0
Vitamin D	0	Vitamin E	0	Pantothenic acid	3	Phosphorus	2
Vitamin K	12	Thiamin	5	Iodine	0	Magnesium	4
Riboflavin	2	Niacin	4	Zinc	2	Selenium	1
Chromium	0	Molybdenum	0	Copper	4	Manganese	15

Lycopene	0 mcg
Omega-3 fatty acids	0 mg
Beta carotene	688 mcg
Lutein/zeaxanthin	108 mcg
Alpha carotene	12 mcg

Flax Meal French Toast

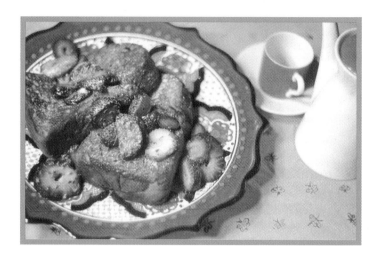

INGREDIENTS

1/4 cup skim milk

2 tbsp. pumpkin butter
(Found in most specialty stores.)

2 egg whites

1 tsp. flax meal

2 slices any whole grain bread

1 cup sliced fruit
(Strawberries or bananas work well.)

1/2 tsp. cinnamon

PREPARATION

1) Mix milk, pumpkin butter, egg whites and
flax meal in a shallow bowl; beat well.

2) Soak the bread in the mixture, turning to soak each side.

3) Place bread in a pan coated with a nonstick spray.

4) Cook on medium heat until lightly browned on both sides.

5) Place sliced fruit on top and sprinkle with cinnamon.

NUTRITION FACTS

Makes 2 servings   Serving size: 1 slice with fruit

Total calories per serving	240	Total protein	10g
Total carbohydrates	45g	Total fat	3.5g
Total fiber	8g	Saturated fat	0.5g

% DAILY REQUIREMENT

Vitamin A	48	Vitamin C	14	Vitamin B_6	11	Folate	14
Calcium	8	Iron	13	Vitamin B_{12}	2	Biotin	0
Vitamin D	0	Vitamin E	0	Pantothenic acid	8	Phosphorus	16
Vitamin K	23	Thiamin	12	Iodine	0	Magnesium	16
Riboflavin	21	Niacin	12	Zinc	8	Selenium	36
Chromium	0	Molybdenum	0	Copper	11	Manganese	70

Lycopene	.17 mcg
Omega-3 fatty acids	640 mg
Beta carotene	24.3 mcg
Lutein/zeaxanthin	102 mcg
Alpha carotene	0 mcg

Oatmeal Pancakes with Bananas

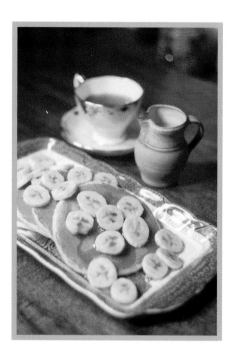

INGREDIENTS

3/4 cup flour

1/4 tsp. baking soda

1 tsp. baking powder

1 tbsp. sugar

1/3 cup quick cooking oats

1/4 tsp. salt

1/4 cup egg substitute or egg whites

2 tbsp. melted butter

1 cup skim milk

1 banana, sliced thinly

PREPARATION

1) Mix flour, baking soda, baking powder, sugar, oats and salt.

2) In another bowl, combine the egg substitute, melted butter and milk.

3) Add the butter and milk mixture to the dry ingredients and mix well.

4) Cook on a heated nonstick skillet.
(Add some nonstick spray if needed.)

5) Place the bananas on top and enjoy!

NUTRITION FACTS

Makes 4 servings   Serving size: 1/4 recipe with fruit

Total calories per serving	240	Total protein	9g
Total carbohydrates	38g	Total fat	6g
Total fiber	3g	Saturated fat	3g

% DAILY REQUIREMENT

Vitamin A	6	Vitamin C	4	Vitamin B$_6$	7	Folate	16
Calcium	24	Iron	13	Vitamin B$_{12}$	6	Biotin	0
Vitamin D	6	Vitamin E	0	Pantothenic acid	10	Phosphorus	32
Vitamin K	1	Thiamin	21	Iodine	0	Magnesium	11
Riboflavin	17	Niacin	9	Zinc	8	Selenium	20
Chromium	0	Molybdenum	0	Copper	7	Manganese	47

Lycopene	0 mcg
Omega-3 fatty acids	100 mg
Beta carotene	49 mcg
Lutein/zeaxanthin	55 mcg
Alpha carotene	6.31 mcg

Blueberry Whole Wheat Waffles

INGREDIENTS

2 low-fat whole wheat waffles, about 1 oz. each

1/2 cup fresh or frozen blueberries

1 tsp. confectioner's sugar

PREPARATION

1) Toast the waffles.

2) Place the blueberries on top of the waffles.

3) Sprinkle with confectioner's sugar.

Note: *You may substitute blueberry preserves (no sugar added) for the sugar. Enjoy with a glass of skim milk.*

NUTRITION FACTS

Makes 1 serving   Serving size: 2 waffles with fruit

Total calories per serving	220	Total protein	5g
Total carbohydrates	44g	Total fat	2.5g
Total fiber	2g	Saturated fat	0.5g

% DAILY REQUIREMENT

Vitamin A	21	Vitamin C	12	Vitamin B$_6$	18	Folate	15
Calcium	4	Iron	23	Vitamin B$_{12}$	18	Biotin	0
Vitamin D	0	Vitamin E	0	Pantothenic acid	1	Phosphorus	7
Vitamin K	17	Thiamin	43	Iodine	0	Magnesium	13
Riboflavin	32	Niacin	27	Zinc	1	Selenium	0
Chromium	0	Molybdenum	0	Copper	2	Manganese	12

Lycopene	0 mcg
Omega-3 fatty acids	40 mg
Beta carotene	23 mcg
Lutein/zeaxanthin	58 mcg
Alpha carotene	0 mcg

Yogurt Treat

INGREDIENTS

1 cup nonfat vanilla yogurt (with live cultures)

1/4 cup sliced blackberries

1/4 cup fresh blueberries

1 tbsp. wheat germ

PREPARATION

Mix yogurt with fruit and wheat germ.

NUTRITION FACTS

Makes 1 serving   Serving size: 1 1/2 cups

Total calories per serving	320	Total protein	15g
Total carbohydrates	63g	Total fat	2g
Total fiber	5g	Saturated fat	0.5g

% DAILY REQUIREMENT

Vitamin A	3	Vitamin C	21	Vitamin B$_6$	16	Folate	18
Calcium	39	Iron	8	Vitamin B$_{12}$	19	Biotin	0
Vitamin D	0	Vitamin E	0	Pantothenic acid	5	Phosphorus	42
Vitamin K	21	Thiamin	26	Iodine	0	Magnesium	20
Riboflavin	32	Niacin	8	Zinc	25	Selenium	37
Chromium	0	Molybdenum	0	Copper	11	Manganese	116

Lycopene	0 mcg
Omega-3 fatty acids	40 mg
Beta carotene	23 mcg
Lutein/zeaxanthin	58 mcg
Alpha carotene	0 mcg

Fruit Wrap

● ● ● ○

INGREDIENTS

1 low carb whole wheat tortilla or crepe

2 tbsp. nonfat vanilla yogurt

1 tbsp. wheat germ

1/4 cup blueberries

1/4 cup sliced strawberries

PREPARATION

1) Heat the tortilla/crepe in a microwave or oven.
(If using the microwave, be sure to heat for only a few seconds.)

2) Spread yogurt on the tortilla/crepe.

3) Sprinkle wheat germ over yogurt.

4) Add fruit and roll up tortilla.

Note: *This is a healthy start to your day.*
Pick any two fruits and any nonfat or low-fat yogurt flavor.

Nutrition Facts

Makes 1 serving   Serving size: 1 fruit wrap

Total calories per serving	170/120	Total protein	10g/7g
Total carbohydrates	33g/23g	Total fat	3.5g/1.5g
Total fiber	12g/5g	Saturated fat	0g/0g

● ●

% Daily Requirement
(Tortilla)

Vitamin A	1	Vitamin C	41	Vitamin B_6	12	Folate	17
Calcium	10	Iron	10	Vitamin B_{12}	2	Biotin	0
Vitamin D	0	Vitamin E	0	Pantothenic acid	4	Phosphorus	17
Vitamin K	10	Thiamin	2	Iodine	1	Magnesium	11
Riboflavin	13	Niacin	8	Zinc	14	Selenium	19
Chromium	0	Molybdenum	0	Copper	8	Manganese	108

% Daily Requirement
(Crepe)

Vitamin A	1	Vitamin C	41	Vitamin B_6	12	Folate	13
Calcium	8	Iron	8	Vitamin B_{12}	2	Biotin	0
Vitamin D	0	Vitamin E	0	Pantothenic acid	4	Phosphorus	17
Vitamin K	10	Thiamin	20	Iodine	0	Magnesium	11
Riboflavin	9	Niacin	6	Zinc	14	Selenium	19
Chromium	0	Molybdenum	0	Copper	8	Manganese	108

(Tortilla/Crepe)

Lycopene	0 mcg
Omega-3 fatty acids	50 mg
Beta carotene	15 mcg
Lutein/zeaxanthin	41 mcg
Alpha carotene	0 mcg

Fruit Mixer

INGREDIENTS

1 orange peeled, sectioned and cut in half

1/2 cup red seedless grapes

1 tbsp. lime juice

1/2 cup cantaloupe melon, cut in small pieces

PREPARATION

Mix all the ingredients together.

Note: *You can substitute any kind of fruit for the melon. Enjoy!*

NUTRITION FACTS

Makes 2 servings   Serving size: 1/2 recipe

Total calories per serving	70	Total protein	1g
Total carbohydrates	19g	Total fat	0g
Total fiber	2g	Saturated fat	0g

% DAILY REQUIREMENT

Vitamin A	31	Vitamin C	93	Vitamin B$_6$	5	Folate	7
Calcium	3	Iron	2	Vitamin B$_{12}$	0	Biotin	0
Vitamin D	0	Vitamin E	0	Pantothenic acid	2	Phosphorus	2
Vitamin K	8	Thiamin	7	Iodine	0	Magnesium	4
Riboflavin	4	Niacin	3	Zinc	1	Selenium	1
Chromium	0	Molybdenum	0	Copper	5	Manganese	3

Lycopene	0 mcg
Omega-3 fatty acids	30 mg
Beta carotene	872 mcg
Lutein/zeaxanthin	123 mcg
Alpha carotene	14 mcg

Egg White Omelet with Salsa & Cheese

INGREDIENTS

3 egg whites

2 tbsp. mild, prepared salsa

(If your family likes it spicy, feel free to use the hot variety.)

1 tbsp. low-fat cheese (any kind you like)

PREPARATION

1) Mix the egg whites with the salsa.

2) Cook the egg mixture in a nonstick skillet.

3) Sprinkle with the cheese.

4) Cook until well done and the cheese has melted.

Note: *You can use any kind of cheese in this recipe. Serve with 1 slice of multi-grain, high-fiber bread & a fruit smoothie (see pages 165-172) for a real treat!*

NUTRITION FACTS

Makes 1 serving   Serving size: 1 omelet

Total calories per serving	100	Total protein	15g
Total carbohydrates	3g	Total fat	3g
Total fiber	0g	Saturated fat	2g

% DAILY REQUIREMENT

Vitamin A	4	Vitamin C	3	Vitamin B$_6$	1	Folate	1
Calcium	12	Iron	1	Vitamin B$_{12}$	7	Biotin	0
Vitamin D	0	Vitamin E	0	Pantothenic acid	2	Phosphorus	9
Vitamin K	0	Thiamin	1	Iodine	0	Magnesium	4
Riboflavin	28	Niacin	1	Zinc	3	Selenium	32
Chromium	0	Molybdenum	0	Copper	0	Manganese	1

Lycopene	0 mcg
Omega-3 fatty acids	30 mg
Beta carotene	6 mcg
Lutein/zeaxanthin	0 mcg
Alpha carotene	0 mcg

Lunch

Caesar Salad

INGREDIENTS

1 tsp. Dijon mustard

1 tbsp. red wine vinegar

1/3 cup extra virgin olive oil

1 clove garlic, minced

1 tbsp. lemon juice

2 tbsp. freshly grated Parmesan cheese

1/4 tsp. salt

1/4 tsp. pepper

1 head of romaine lettuce, leaves individually washed

Handful of shaved Parmesan cheese

PREPARATION

1) Mix mustard, vinegar, oil, garlic, lemon juice,
grated Parmesan cheese, salt and pepper.

2) Cut the lettuce leaves into bite size pieces and mix with dressing.

3) Sprinkle with Parmesan shavings.

Note: *Caesar salad contains a high amount of calories from fat.*
The fat is mainly derived from monounsaturated fats from the olive oil
and can be used as your added fat allotment for the day.

NUTRITION FACTS

Makes 4 servings   *Serving size: ¹/4 recipe*

Total calories per serving	140	Total protein	2g
Total carbohydrates	4g	Total fat	13g
Total fiber	2g	Saturated fat	2g

% DAILY REQUIREMENT

Vitamin A	121	Vitamin C	43	Vitamin B_6	4	Folate	36
Calcium	6	Iron	7	Vitamin B_{12}	1	Biotin	0
Vitamin D	0	Vitamin E	0	Pantothenic acid	2	Phosphorus	5
Vitamin K	143	Thiamin	5	Iodine	0	Magnesium	4
Riboflavin	5	Niacin	2	Zinc	2	Selenium	2
Chromium	0	Molybdenum	0	Copper	3	Manganese	9

Lycopene	0 mcg
Omega-3 fatty acids	230 mg
Beta carotene	3636 mcg
Lutein/zeaxanthin	2415 mcg
Alpha carotene	0 mcg

Salad in a Pita

INGREDIENTS

1/4 cup toasted walnuts

*(To toast walnuts, place them on a nonstick pan and heat
in 350° oven until lightly browned.)*

1/2 orange, peeled and cut

1 tsp. dried cranberries

2 leaves of romaine lettuce, washed and cut

3 slices deli turkey, cut into thin strips

1 tbsp. low-fat balsamic vinaigrette dressing

1 small, whole wheat pita bread

PREPARATION

1) Mix together walnuts, orange, cranberries and dressing.

2) Toss with lettuce and turkey.

3) Slice open pita and place salad ingredients inside.

Note: *This is a healthy lunch to take to work or school.
(Add the dressing just before eating.)*

NUTRITION FACTS

Makes 1 serving   Serving size: 1 sandwich

Total calories per serving	260	Total protein	22g
Total carbohydrates	27g	Total fat	9g
Total fiber	5g	Saturated fat	1g

· ·

% DAILY REQUIREMENT

Vitamin A	17	Vitamin C	64	Vitamin B$_6$	8	Folate	13
Calcium	4	Iron	7	Vitamin B$_{12}$	0	Biotin	0
Vitamin D	0	Vitamin E	0	Pantothenic acid	5	Phosphorus	9
Vitamin K	18	Thiamin	12	Iodine	0	Magnesium	10
Riboflavin	4	Niacin	6	Zinc	5	Selenium	19
Chromium	0	Molybdenum	0	Copper	12	Manganese	39

Lycopene	0 mcg
Omega-3 fatty acids	870 mg
Beta carotene	466 mcg
Lutein/zeaxanthin	380 mcg
Alpha carotene	7 mcg

Single Serving Easy Pizza

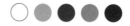

INGREDIENTS

1 whole wheat wrap

$1/2$ cup tomato sauce

1 oz. low-fat shredded mozzarella cheese

$1/4$ cup sliced peppers, any color

$1/4$ cup sliced mushrooms

PREPARATION

1) Warm the wrap in a 350° oven, but do not let it toast. (You may use pita bread instead of a wrap.)

2) Remove wrap from the oven and spread with tomato sauce.

3) Sprinkle with the cheese and any other vegetable toppings.

4) Put back in the oven until the cheese is melted.

Note: *Tomato sauce is very healthy so be generous! You can add any other vegetables as toppings.*

Nutrition Facts

Makes 1 serving   Serving size: 1 small pizza

Total calories per serving   220   Total protein   13g

Total carbohydrates   29g   Total fat   7g

Total fiber   5g   Saturated fat   3.5g

% Daily Requirement

Vitamin A	26	Vitamin C	90	Vitamin B$_6$	16	Folate	9
Calcium	23	Iron	16	Vitamin B$_{12}$	11	Biotin	0
Vitamin D	0	Vitamin E	0	Pantothenic acid	16	Phosphorus	27
Vitamin K	7	Thiamin	13	Iodine	0	Magnesium	13
Riboflavin	20	Niacin	20	Zinc	13	Selenium	31
Chromium	0	Molybdenum	0	Copper	22	Manganese	35

Lycopene	18,632 mcg
Omega-3 fatty acids	80 mg
Beta carotene	642 mcg
Lutein/zeaxanthin	27 mcg
Alpha carotene	5 mcg

Grilled Tofu & Tomato Sandwich

INGREDIENTS

Dijon mustard

2 slices whole grain bread, toasted

3 slices of medium tofu, about 1/2" thick
(Note: medium refers to the texture of the tofu.)

3 thick slices tomato

PREPARATION

1) Spread mustard on both slices of bread.

2) Place the tofu on the bread and then place the tomatoes on top.

3) Prepare a skillet with a little canola oil or nonstick spray; toast the sandwich until golden brown on both sides.

NUTRITION FACTS

Makes 1 serving   Serving size: 1 sandwich

Total calories per serving	260	Total protein	23g
Total carbohydrates	33g	Total fat	6g
Total fiber	5g	Saturated fat	1g

% DAILY REQUIREMENT

Vitamin A	8	Vitamin C	26	Vitamin B$_6$	8	Folate	10
Calcium	15	Iron	24	Vitamin B$_{12}$	0	Biotin	0
Vitamin D	0	Vitamin E	0	Pantothenic acid	5	Phosphorus	37
Vitamin K	2	Thiamin	23	Iodine	0	Magnesium	22
Riboflavin	12	Niacin	15	Zinc	14	Selenium	36
Chromium	0	Molybdenum	0	Copper	26	Manganese	71

Lycopene	0 mcg
Omega-3 fatty acids	120 mg
Beta carotene	2.34 mcg
Lutein/zeaxanthin	53 mcg
Alpha carotene	0 mcg

Dinner

Turkey Meatballs

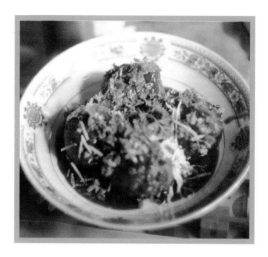

INGREDIENTS

1 cup onions, chopped

1 cup chicken broth

1 lb. lean turkey, ground

1 cup Italian seasoned bread crumbs

1 egg

2 cups tomato sauce

Salt and pepper to taste

PREPARATION

1) Sauté the onions in 1-2 tablespoons of chicken broth until lightly browned.

2) In a large mixing bowl combine the turkey, bread crumbs and sautéed onions.

3) Beat the egg and add to turkey mixture.

4) Slowly add some broth until the mixture feels moist.
(You may need to adjust the broth amount so the mixture doesn't get too soggy.)

5) Form into balls and place on a baking pan
sprayed with nonstick spray.

6) Place into a pre-heated 350° oven and bake for 45-60 minutes
until well cooked and browned on the outside.

7) Pour sauce over meatballs and serve!

Nutrition Facts

Makes 4 servings   Serving size: 1/4 recipe

Total calories per serving	280	Total protein	25g
Total carbohydrates	20g	Total fat	12g
Total fiber	3g	Saturated fat	3g

% Daily Requirement

Vitamin A	10	Vitamin C	19	Vitamin B_6	30	Folate	11
Calcium	6	Iron	19	Vitamin B_{12}	10	Biotin	0
Vitamin D	1	Vitamin E	0	Pantothenic acid	14	Phosphorus	27
Vitamin K	6	Thiamin	11	Iodine	0	Magnesium	12
Riboflavin	20	Niacin	32	Zinc	18	Selenium	41
Chromium	0	Molybdenum	0	Copper	16	Manganese	13

Lycopene	18,561 mcg
Omega-3 fatty acids	160 mg
Beta carotene	258 mcg
Lutein/zeaxanthin	43 mcg
Alpha carotene	0 mcg

Bean Tacos

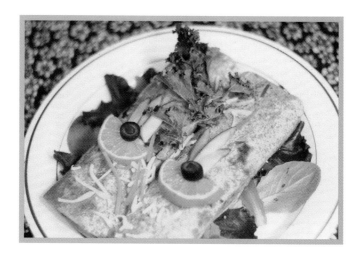

INGREDIENTS

1 16-oz. can pinto beans

1 cup salsa, mild or hot

Chili powder, to taste

2 large whole wheat tortillas

$^1/_2$ cup shredded Mexican blend mixed cheese

PREPARATION

1) Heat the pinto beans until soft and mash them in a bowl.

2) Add the salsa and season with chili powder.

3) Line the tortillas with the bean mixture,
sprinkle with cheese and roll into a taco.

NUTRITION FACTS

Makes 2 servings   *Serving size: 1 taco*

Total calories per serving	410	Total protein	24g
Total carbohydrates	65g	Total fat	7g
Total fiber	16g	Saturated fat	2g

% DAILY REQUIREMENT

Vitamin A	18	Vitamin C	17	Vitamin B$_6$	7	Folate	41
Calcium	25	Iron	26	Vitamin B$_{12}$	2	Biotin	0
Vitamin D	0	Vitamin E	0	Pantothenic acid	5	Phosphorus	40
Vitamin K	10	Thiamin	32	Iodine	0	Magnesium	20
Riboflavin	23	Niacin	14	Zinc	13	Selenium	24
Chromium	0	Molybdenum	0	Copper	20	Manganese	40

Lycopene	0.27 mcg
Omega-3 fatty acids	310 mg
Beta carotene	196 mcg
Lutein/zeaxanthin	10 mcg
Alpha carotene	27 mcg

Broccoli & Turkey Teriyaki Stir Fry

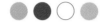

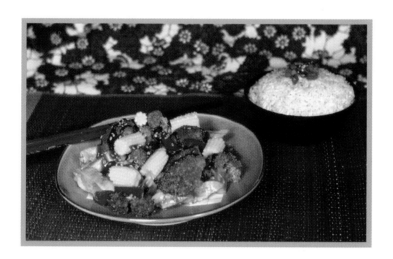

INGREDIENTS

2 tbsp. canola oil

4 turkey cutlets, sliced into thin strips

3 tbsp. soy sauce

1 bunch broccoli, cut up

1 red pepper, cut into small pieces

1 cup baby corn (canned is fine)

1 tsp. teriyaki sauce

4 cups brown rice, cooked

PREPARATION

1) Coat a wok or large frying pan with
1 tablespoon canola oil and heat.

2) Add turkey strips, 1 tablespoon soy sauce and cook
until the turkey is cooked through.

3) Remove turkey from the pan with a slotted spoon.

4) Add the vegetables, remaining soy sauce and teriyaki sauce; stir fry until vegetables are slightly tender.

(Increase or decrease the amount of soy sauce to taste.)

5) Add the turkey back to the wok and quickly stir to heat the turkey.

6) Serve over brown rice.

NUTRITION FACTS

Makes 4 servings   Serving size: 1/4 recipe

Total calories per serving	570	Total protein	43g
Total carbohydrates	66g	Total fat	16g
Total fiber	9g	Saturated fat	3.5g

% DAILY REQUIREMENT

Vitamin A	39	Vitamin C	325	Vitamin B_6	57	Folate	35
Calcium	14	Iron	27	Vitamin B_{12}	8	Biotin	0
Vitamin D	0	Vitamin E	0	Pantothenic acid	37	Phosphorus	51
Vitamin K	197	Thiamin	30	Iodine	0	Magnesium	42
Riboflavin	30	Niacin	46	Zinc	43	Selenium	72
Chromium	0	Molybdenum	0	Copper	24	Manganese	132

Lycopene	92 mcg
Omega-3 fatty acids	510 mg
Beta carotene	1066 mcg
Lutein/zeaxanthin	2599 mcg
Alpha carotene	44 mcg

Soft Tacos with Lentils & Veggies

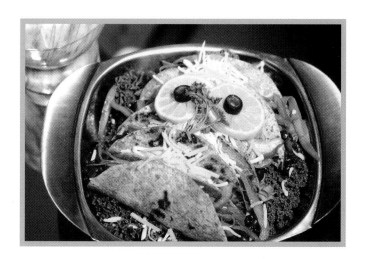

INGREDIENTS

1 cup dry lentils

3 cups water

1 tbsp. olive oil

3 carrots, cut into thin slices

2 green peppers, cut into thin strips

1 cup mild salsa

4 small, whole wheat tortillas

1 cup low-fat, shredded Mexican blend mixed cheese

PREPARATION

1) Bring the water to a boil, add lentils and
cook until soft (about 30 minutes).

2) Drain lentils and set aside.

3) Coat frying pan with olive oil and sauté carrots and pepper until soft.

4) Stir in the salsa.

5) Add the vegetable mixture to the lentils and stir until well mixed.

6) Scoop mixture into the tortillas.
Sprinkle the cheese on top and serve.

NUTRITION FACTS

Makes 4 servings   Serving size: 1 taco

Total calories per serving	430	Total protein	26g
Total carbohydrates	56g	Total fat	13g
Total fiber	18g	Saturated fat	5g

% DAILY REQUIREMENT

Vitamin A	123	Vitamin C	302	Vitamin B_6	26	Folate	69
Calcium	30	Iron	34	Vitamin B_{12}	4	Biotin	0
Vitamin D	0	Vitamin E	0	Pantothenic acid	12	Phosphorus	42
Vitamin K	15	Thiamin	30	Iodine	0	Magnesium	21
Riboflavin	21	Niacin	18	Zinc	20	Selenium	21
Chromium	0	Molybdenum	0	Copper	29	Manganese	50

Lycopene	0 mcg
Omega-3 fatty acids	80 mg
Beta carotene	342 mcg
Lutein/zeaxanthin	154 mcg
Alpha carotene	150 mcg

Vegetarian Chili

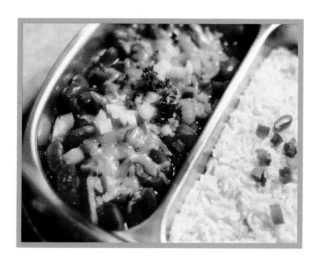

INGREDIENTS

2 large carrots, thinly sliced

1 large white onion, finely chopped

2 large celery sticks, thinly sliced

1 orange bell pepper, core removed and diced

1 clove garlic, finely minced

2 tbsp. extra virgin olive oil

2 16-oz. cans drained kidney beans

2 cups canned chopped tomatoes

2 cups chicken broth

1 tsp. cumin

1 tbsp. chili powder

$1/2$ tsp. salt

1 tbsp. low-fat cheddar cheese, grated

PREPARATION

1) Sauté carrots, onions, celery, pepper and garlic in olive oil
in a large pot until all ingredients are tender.

2) Add the beans, chopped tomatoes (including the liquid),
chicken broth, cumin, chili powder and salt
(adjust the amount of seasoning to taste).

3) Simmer on low heat for 30-40 minutes, stirring occasionally.

4) Pour into bowls and sprinkle with 1 tablespoon low-fat cheddar cheese.

5) Serve with whole wheat pita bread.

NUTRITION FACTS

Makes 4 servings   Serving size: 1 cup

Total calories per serving	330	Total protein	16g
Total carbohydrates	48g	Total fat	9g
Total fiber	13g	Saturated fat	1.5g

% DAILY REQUIREMENT

Vitamin A	39	Vitamin C	94	Vitamin B_6	30	Folate	29
Calcium	15	Iron	26	Vitamin B_{12}	1	Biotin	0
Vitamin D	0	Vitamin E	0	Pantothenic acid	5	Phosphorus	30
Vitamin K	39	Thiamin	26	Iodine	0	Magnesium	25
Riboflavin	15	Niacin	18	Zinc	11	Selenium	5
Chromium	0	Molybdenum	0	Copper	32	Manganese	31

Lycopene	12,291 mcg
Omega-3 fatty acids	120 mg
Beta carotene	685 mcg
Lutein/zeaxanthin	170 mcg
Alpha carotene	157 mcg

Sautéed Shrimp & Beans

INGREDIENTS

2 tbsp. olive oil

1 small onion, chopped

2 cloves garlic, minced

1 cup green pepper, chopped

1 lb. medium shrimp, cleaned and deveined

1 tsp. salt

$1/4$ tsp. pepper

1 tsp. Italian seasoning

$1/2$ cup fresh or canned tomatoes, chopped

1 can pinto beans, rinsed and drained

2 cups brown rice

PREPARATION

1) Sauté onions and garlic in olive oil; add the green pepper.

2) Add shrimp, salt, pepper and Italian seasoning,
and cook until shrimp are pink on both sides.
(This only takes a few minutes.)

3) Quickly add the tomatoes and beans and stir together.

4) Serve over brown rice.

NUTRITION FACTS

Makes 4 servings   Serving size: ¹/4 recipe

Total calories per serving	400	Total protein	32g
Total carbohydrates	46g	Total fat	10g
Total fiber	8g	Saturated fat	1.5g

% DAILY REQUIREMENT

Vitamin A	11	Vitamin C	69	Vitamin B$_6$	27	Folate	22
Calcium	11	Iron	33	Vitamin B$_{12}$	28	Biotin	0
Vitamin D	0	Vitamin E	0	Pantothenic acid	11	Phosphorus	35
Vitamin K	12	Thiamin	20	Iodine	0	Magnesium	30
Riboflavin	9	Niacin	25	Zinc	22	Selenium	76
Chromium	0	Molybdenum	0	Copper	25	Manganese	75

Lycopene	0 mcg
Omega-3 fatty acids	610 mg
Beta carotene	78 mcg
Lutein/zeaxanthin	129 mcg
Alpha carotene	7.9 mcg

Noodles with Peanut Butter Sauce

INGREDIENTS

1 15-oz. can of cooked peas
(Or use frozen or fresh.)

1/2 lb. whole wheat pasta (any type)

1/3 cup peanut butter
(Be sure to use peanut butter with no added sugar.)

2 cloves garlic

2 tbsp. soy sauce

2/3 cup chicken broth

1 1/2 tbsp. lime juice

1/2 tsp. salt

PREPARATION

1) Drain the peas and put aside.

2) Cook the pasta until al dente.

3) Mix the remaining ingredients in a blender until smooth.

4) Combine the peanut sauce with the pasta and then add the peas.

5) Mix well and serve.

NUTRITION FACTS

Makes 4 servings   Serving size: ¹/4 recipe

Total calories per serving	350	Total protein	17g
Total carbohydrates	51g	Total fat	12g
Total fiber	2g	Saturated fat	2.5g

• •

% DAILY REQUIREMENT

Vitamin A	1	Vitamin C	3	Vitamin B_6	17	Folate	15
Calcium	4	Iron	17	Vitamin B_{12}	1	Biotin	0
Vitamin D	0	Vitamin E	0	Pantothenic acid	9	Phosphorus	27
Vitamin K	0	Thiamin	22	Iodine	0	Magnesium	31
Riboflavin	9	Niacin	35	Zinc	15	Selenium	61
Chromium	0	Molybdenum	0	Copper	21	Manganese	110

Lycopene	0 mcg
Omega-3 fatty acids	20 mg
Beta carotene	0 mcg
Lutein/zeaxanthin	0.19 mcg
Alpha carotene	0 mcg

Shrimp & Oranges over Pasta

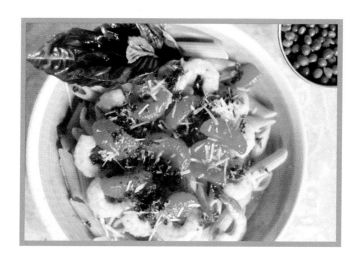

INGREDIENTS

$1/2$ lb. whole wheat penne pasta

1 small white onion, minced

1 tbsp. olive oil

$1/2$ lb. small shrimp, cleaned and deveined

$1/4$ cup chicken broth

$1/2$ tsp. orange peel, freshly grated

Salt to taste

Dash of pepper

2 fresh oranges, peeled and sliced

Romano cheese, to taste

PREPARATION

1) Cook the pasta until al dente.

2) Sauté onion in the olive oil until slightly browned.

3) Mix in the shrimp, chicken broth, orange peel,

pepper and salt to taste.

4) Sauté until shrimp turn pink.

5) Toss the shrimp mixture over cooked pasta; mix in the orange slices.

6) Sprinkle with Romano cheese.

NUTRITION FACTS

Makes 4 servings   Serving size: 1/4 recipe

Total calories per serving	330	Total protein	21g
Total carbohydrates	53g	Total fat	5g
Total fiber	2g	Saturated fat	1g

% DAILY REQUIREMENT

Vitamin A	5	Vitamin C	62	Vitamin B$_6$	13	Folate	14
Calcium	8	Iron	20	Vitamin B$_{12}$	11	Biotin	0
Vitamin D	22	Vitamin E	0	Pantothenic acid	9	Phosphorus	28
Vitamin K	3	Thiamin	24	Iodine	0	Magnesium	28
Riboflavin	8	Niacin	23	Zinc	14	Selenium	91
Chromium	0	Molybdenum	0	Copper	22	Manganese	90

Lycopene	0 mcg
Omega-3 fatty acids	310 mg
Beta carotene	47 mcg
Lutein/zeaxanthin	85 mcg
Alpha carotene	7.21 mcg

Vegetable Rolls

INGREDIENTS

4 whole wheat lasagna noodles, cooked

1 clove garlic, chopped

1 tbsp. olive oil

1 cup cooked and drained spinach/kale

1 cup cooked carrots, cut into small pieces

Salt and pepper to taste

1/2 cup part-skim shredded mozzarella cheese

1 cup part-skim ricotta cheese

2 cups tomato sauce

PREPARATION

1) Cook the lasagna as directed on the package.

2) When cooked, lay out each noodle on a moist towel
to keep it from drying out.

3) Sauté the garlic in olive oil; add the spinach and carrots and mix quickly.

4) Add the salt and pepper to taste.

5) Add mozzarella and ricotta cheese to the vegetable mixture.

6) Divide mixture into 4 portions and spread one portion on each lasagna noodle. Gently roll up the noodle. Repeat filling the other noodles.

7) Place the lasagna rolls, seam down, in a lasagna pan and pour tomato sauce over them.

8) Bake in 400° oven until cheese is melted.

Note: *You can add 4 ounces of cooked, chopped turkey meat to this recipe for added protein.*

NUTRITION FACTS

Makes 4 servings   Serving size: 1 roll

Total calories per serving	270	Total protein	16g
Total carbohydrates	35g	Total fat	7g
Total fiber	4g	Saturated fat	4g

% DAILY REQUIREMENT

Vitamin A	117	Vitamin C	37	Vitamin B_6	1	Folate	2
Calcium	30	Iron	12	Vitamin B_{12}	3	Biotin	0
Vitamin D	0	Vitamin E	0	Pantothenic acid	2	Phosphorus	16
Vitamin K	0	Thiamin	19	Iodine	0	Magnesium	2
Riboflavin	16	Niacin	8	Zinc	8	Selenium	15
Chromium	0	Molybdenum	0	Copper	1	Manganese	1

Lycopene	0 mcg
Omega-3 fatty acids	40 mg
Beta carotene	2656 mcg
Lutein/zeaxanthin	5930 mcg
Alpha carotene	0 mcg

Chicken & Green Stir Fry

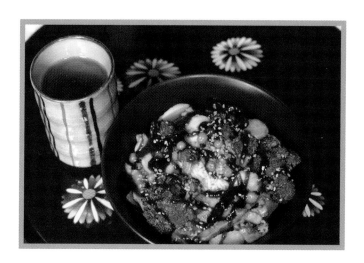

INGREDIENTS

1/4 cup onion, chopped

2 tbsp. sesame oil

1 lb. thin chicken cutlet, cut into skinny strips

1 cup peas, frozen

1 cup broccoli, chopped

1/2 cup water chestnuts, sliced

2 tbsp. soy sauce

2 cups cold brown rice

Preparation

1) Sauté the onions in 1 tablespoon of sesame oil in
a skillet or wok, and cook until onions are clear.

2) Add the chicken and cook until almost done.

3) Add the peas, broccoli and water chestnuts; mix in soy sauce.

4) Stir fry until and all the ingredients are cooked through.

5) Stir in rice until warmed.

Nutrition Facts

Makes 4 servings   Serving size: 1/4 recipe

Total calories per serving	330	Total protein	31g
Total carbohydrates	33g	Total fat	12g
Total fiber	5g	Saturated fat	2g

% Daily Requirement

Vitamin A	9	Vitamin C	29	Vitamin B$_6$	33	Folate	4
Calcium	3	Iron	11	Vitamin B$_{12}$	7	Biotin	0
Vitamin D	0	Vitamin E	0	Pantothenic acid	16	Phosphorus	28
Vitamin K	1	Thiamin	13	Iodine	0	Magnesium	18
Riboflavin	10	Niacin	53	Zinc	16	Selenium	26
Chromium	0	Molybdenum	0	Copper	8	Manganese	56

Lycopene	0 mcg
Omega-3 fatty acids	70 mg
Beta carotene	0 mcg
Lutein/zeaxanthin	0 mcg
Alpha carotene	0 mcg

Whole Wheat Penne with Cauliflower

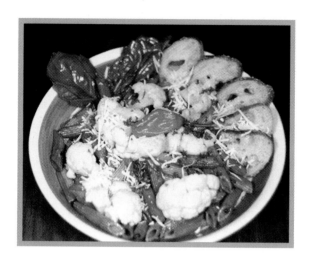

INGREDIENTS

1 head of cauliflower, washed and separated

1 onion, chopped

3 cloves garlic, chopped

2 tbsp. extra virgin olive oil

Salt and pepper taste

1/2 lb. whole wheat penne pasta

3 tsp. Parmesan cheese, grated

PREPARATION

1) Steam the cauliflower florets until soft.

2) Boil the pasta according to the directions on the package.

3) Sauté onions and garlic in the olive oil.

4) Add the cauliflower and mix until coated with olive oil;
cook on low heat.

5) Add salt and pepper to taste.

6) Combine penne with the cauliflower; toss until coated.

7) Sprinkle 3/4 teaspoon Parmesan cheese on each serving.

NUTRITION FACTS

Makes 4 servings   Serving size: 1/4 recipe

Total calories per serving	330	Total protein	16g
Total carbohydrates	42g	Total fat	11g
Total fiber	10g	Saturated fat	2.5g

% DAILY REQUIREMENT

Vitamin A	5	Vitamin C	17	Vitamin B_6	15	Folate	17
Calcium	17	Iron	2	Vitamin B_{12}	2	Biotin	0
Vitamin D	0	Vitamin E	22	Pantothenic acid	9	Phosphorus	14
Vitamin K	3	Thiamin	27	Iodine	0	Magnesium	7
Riboflavin	13	Niacin	15	Zinc	7	Selenium	4
Chromium	0	Molybdenum	0	Copper	3	Manganese	16

Lycopene	0 mcg
Omega-3 fatty acids	0 mg
Beta carotene	0 mcg
Lutein/zeaxanthin	0 mcg
Alpha carotene	0 mcg

Chicken Strips
A Great Substitute for Chicken Nuggets

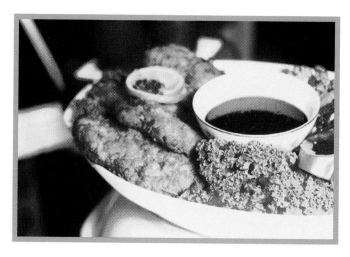

INGREDIENTS

2 cups ground Golden Flax™ cereal
(or any other high-fiber cereal)

2 tbsp. wheat germ

Salt and pepper to taste

1 egg, large

1 lb. chicken breast cutlets, cut into long, thin strips

2 tbsp. olive oil

PREPARATION

1) Combine the cereal, wheat germ, salt and pepper in a bowl.

2) Beat the egg in another bowl.
(Add a little water if it is too thick.)

3) Dip each chicken strip into the egg and then into the cereal.

4) Heat the olive oil and cook the chicken strips over medium heat, turning to cook both sides, until well done.

Nutrition Facts

Makes 4 servings   Serving size: 4 oz. or ¼ recipe

Total calories per serving	310	Total protein	16g
Total carbohydrates	16g	Total fat	11g
Total fiber	4g	Saturated fat	2.5g

% Daily Requirement

Vitamin A	2	Vitamin C	2	Vitamin B_6	32	Folate	5
Calcium	2	Iron	7	Vitamin B_{12}	10	Biotin	0
Vitamin D	1	Vitamin E	0	Pantothenic acid	11	Phosphorus	25
Vitamin K	0	Thiamin	11	Iodine	0	Magnesium	11
Riboflavin	12	Niacin	65	Zinc	7	Selenium	35
Chromium	0	Molybdenum	0	Copper	3	Manganese	1

Lycopene	0 mcg
Omega-3 fatty acids	40 mg
Beta carotene	1 mcg
Lutein/zeaxanthin	48 mcg
Alpha carotene	0 mcg

Grilled Salmon

INGREDIENTS

1/2 cup bread crumbs

2 cups canned crushed tomatoes, undrained

Salt and pepper to taste

1 tbsp. Italian seasoning

1 lb. fresh, non-farmed salmon

PREPARATION

1) Mix together bread crumbs, tomatoes, salt, pepper and Italian seasoning.

2) Spread evenly over salmon.

3) Place in a nonstick baking dish and cook at 375° for about 30 minutes, until completely cooked.

NUTRITION FACTS

Makes 4 serving   Serving size: 1/4 recipe

Total calories per serving	170	Total protein	24g
Total carbohydrates	8g	Total fat	4.5g
Total fiber	1g	Saturated fat	0.5g

% DAILY REQUIREMENT

Vitamin A	6	Vitamin C	19	Vitamin B$_6$	17	Folate	5
Calcium	6	Iron	14	Vitamin B$_{12}$	57	Biotin	0
Vitamin D	0	Vitamin E	0	Pantothenic acid	11	Phosphorus	29
Vitamin K	11	Thiamin	18	Iodine	0	Magnesium	11
Riboflavin	9	Niacin	45	Zinc	6	Selenium	75
Chromium	0	Molybdenum	0	Copper	9	Manganese	8

Lycopene	3241 mcg
Omega-3 fatty acids	1190 mg
Beta carotene	101 mcg
Lutein/zeaxanthin	116 mcg
Alpha carotene	5 mcg

Smoothies

Banana Cherry Smoothie

INGREDIENTS

1/2 cup frozen cherries

1 cup skim milk

2 tbsp. toasted wheat germ

1/2 banana, sliced

2 tbsp. honey

1/2 cup chopped ice

PREPARATION

Combine all ingredients in a blender until smooth.

NUTRITION FACTS

Makes 2 servings   Serving size: 1/2 recipe

Total calories per serving	170	Total protein	7g
Total carbohydrates	79g	Total fat	1g
Total fiber	2g	Saturated fat	0g

% DAILY REQUIREMENT

Vitamin A	7	Vitamin C	7	Vitamin B$_6$	12	Folate	3
Calcium	15	Iron	5	Vitamin B$_{12}$	8	Biotin	0
Vitamin D	0	Vitamin E	0	Pantothenic acid	1	Phosphorus	12
Vitamin K	0	Thiamin	12	Iodine	0	Magnesium	6
Riboflavin	16	Niacin	3	Zinc	3	Selenium	3
Chromium	0	Molybdenum	8	Copper	4	Manganese	4

Lycopene	0 mcg
Omega-3 fatty acids	0 mg
Beta carotene	0 mcg
Lutein/zeaxanthin	0 mcg
Alpha carotene	0 mcg

Wheat Germ & Fruit Smoothie

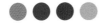

INGREDIENTS

1 cup fresh orange juice, with pulp

1/2 cup blueberries, fresh or frozen

2 tbsp. toasted wheat germ

1 cup canned pear halves in light syrup, drained

Ice cubes, to make shake thick

PREPARATION

Mix all ingredients in blender until well blended and thick.

Note: *You may have to add more ice or orange juice to adjust the consistency if it's too thick.*

NUTRITION FACTS

Makes 2 servings   Serving size: 1/2 recipe

Total calories per serving	170	Total protein	3g
Total carbohydrates	40g	Total fat	1g
Total fiber	2g	Saturated fat	0g

% DAILY REQUIREMENT

Vitamin A	0	Vitamin C	77	Vitamin B$_6$	0	Folate	8
Calcium	1	Iron	3	Vitamin B$_{12}$	0	Biotin	0
Vitamin D	0	Vitamin E	0	Pantothenic acid	0	Phosphorus	8
Vitamin K	9	Thiamin	6	Iodine	0	Magnesium	6
Riboflavin	1	Niacin	3	Zinc	0	Selenium	0
Chromium	0	Molybdenum	0	Copper	1	Manganese	0

Lycopene	0 mcg
Omega-3 fatty acids	20 mg
Beta carotene	0 mcg
Lutein/zeaxanthin	29 mcg
Alpha carotene	0 mcg

Chocolate Peanut Butter Smoothie

INGREDIENTS

3/4 cup low-fat chocolate soy milk

3/4 tbsp. natural peanut butter (no added sugar)

1/2 cup crushed ice

PREPARATION

Mix all ingredients in blender until well blended and thick.

Note: *This is a great snack!*

NUTRITION FACTS

Makes 1 serving   Serving size: 1 recipe

Total calories per serving	160	Total protein	5g
Total carbohydrates	20g	Total fat	8g
Total fiber	2g	Saturated fat	1.5g

% DAILY REQUIREMENT

Vitamin A	8	Vitamin C	0	Vitamin B$_6$	0	Folate	0
Calcium	22	Iron	9	Vitamin B$_{12}$	0	Biotin	0
Vitamin D	19	Vitamin E	0	Pantothenic acid	0	Phosphorus	19
Vitamin K	0	Thiamin	0	Iodine	0	Magnesium	8
Riboflavin	19	Niacin	8	Zinc	0	Selenium	0
Chromium	0	Molybdenum	0	Copper	1	Manganese	0

Lycopene	0 mcg
Omega-3 fatty acids	0 mg
Beta carotene	0 mcg
Lutein/zeaxanthin	0 mcg
Alpha carotene	0 mcg

Almond Strawberry Smoothie

INGREDIENTS

1 cup skim milk

2 tbsp. honey

1 tbsp. toasted almonds, chopped

4 oz. strawberries (frozen work better)

1/2 cup crushed ice cubes

PREPARATION

Combine all ingredients in a blender until smooth.

Note: *This smoothie can be enjoyed as a snack or a dessert!*

NUTRITION FACTS

Makes 2 servings   Serving size: 1/2 recipe

Total calories per serving	160	Total protein	6g
Total carbohydrates	29g	Total fat	3.5g
Total fiber	2g	Saturated fat	0g

% DAILY REQUIREMENT

Vitamin A	6	Vitamin C	39	Vitamin B_6	3	Folate	4
Calcium	19	Iron	4	Vitamin B_{12}	11	Biotin	0
Vitamin D	13	Vitamin E	0	Pantothenic acid	5	Phosphorus	13
Vitamin K	0	Thiamin	5	Iodine	0	Magnesium	5
Riboflavin	17	Niacin	3	Zinc	4	Selenium	6
Chromium	0	Molybdenum	0	Copper	3	Manganese	8

Lycopene	0 mcg
Omega-3 fatty acids	15 mg
Beta carotene	15 mcg
Lutein/zeaxanthin	15 mcg
Alpha carotene	0 mcg

Banana & Strawberry Tofu Smoothie

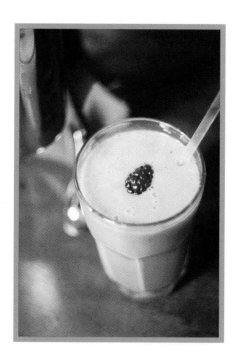

INGREDIENTS

1 banana

1 cup strawberries

3 tbsp. honey

3 oz. soft tofu, drained

1 tsp. walnuts

1/4 tsp. vanilla extract

1/2 cup crushed ice

PREPARATION

Combine all ingredients in a blender until smooth.

Note: *You may have to vary the amount of ice, but start with a small handful.*

NUTRITION FACTS

Makes 2 servings   Serving size: ¹/₂ recipe

Total calories per serving	220	Total protein	3g
Total carbohydrates	50g	Total fat	2.5g
Total fiber	5g	Saturated fat	0g

% DAILY REQUIREMENT

Vitamin A	2	Vitamin C	44	Vitamin B_6	17	Folate	3
Calcium	4	Iron	7	Vitamin B_{12}	0	Biotin	0
Vitamin D	0	Vitamin E	0	Pantothenic acid	2	Phosphorus	2
Vitamin K	0	Thiamin	5	Iodine	0	Magnesium	5
Riboflavin	4	Niacin	2	Zinc	1	Selenium	1
Chromium	0	Molybdenum	0	Copper	4	Manganese	7

Lycopene	0 mcg
Omega-3 fatty acids	35 mg
Beta carotene	45 mcg
Lutein/zeaxanthin	42 mcg
Alpha carotene	15 mcg

Snacks

Spinach Dip with Chips

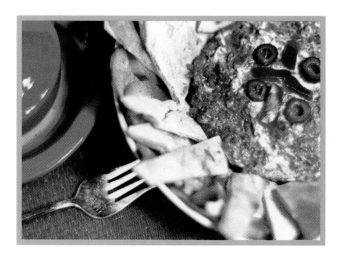

INGREDIENTS

2 cups spinach, cooked

$1/4$ cup skim milk

$1/2$ cup onion, finely chopped

1 tbsp. extra virgin olive oil

1 tbsp. flour

$1/2$ cup low-fat mozzarella cheese, shredded

PREPARATION

1) Drain excess water from spinach.

2) Chop the spinach and mix with $1/2$ cup of the milk. Set aside.

3) Sauté the onions in the olive oil until soft and clear.

4) Add flour and $1/4$ cup of milk, and sauté on low until the sauce thickens.

5) Remove from heat and add the cheese; stir until melted.

6) Immediately combine the spinach/milk mixture.

7) Serve with whole wheat pita chips.

Nutrition Facts

Makes 4 servings   Serving size: $1/4$ recipe

Total calories per serving	120	Total protein	9g
Total carbohydrates	8g	Total fat	4.5g
Total fiber	3g	Saturated fat	0.5g

% Daily Requirement

Vitamin A	362	Vitamin C	17	Vitamin B_6	2	Folate	0
Calcium	20	Iron	4	Vitamin B_{12}	48	Biotin	0
Vitamin D	0	Vitamin E	0	Pantothenic acid	0	Phosphorus	5
Vitamin K	0	Thiamin	2	Iodine	3	Magnesium	1
Riboflavin	5	Niacin	1	Zinc	1	Selenium	1
Chromium	0	Molybdenum	0	Copper	1	Manganese	0

Lycopene	0 mcg
Omega-3 fatty acids	0 mg
Beta carotene	21 mcg
Lutein/zeaxanthin	87 mcg
Alpha carotene	0 mcg

Hummus

INGREDIENTS

1 19-oz. can chick peas, drained and rinsed

1 large clove garlic, finely chopped

1/8 cup tahini
(a paste made from ground sesame seed)

1/8 cup lemon juice

1/4 cup chicken broth

1/4 tsp. cumin

Note: *Tahini can be purchased at many convenience stores.*

PREPARATION

1) Mix in a blender all ingredients except for the chicken broth.

2) When the mixture is blended, gradually add the chicken broth.

3) Add more or less cumin, to taste.

4) Continue to mix until thick and creamy.

5) Serve in a bowl with wedges of whole wheat pita bread.

Nutrition Facts

Makes 4 servings   *Serving size: 1/4 recipe*

Total calories per serving	160	Total protein	7g
Total carbohydrates	18g	Total fat	7g
Total fiber	4g	Saturated fat	0g

% Daily Requirement

Vitamin A	0	Vitamin C	3	Vitamin B_6	1	Folate	2
Calcium	6	Iron	14	Vitamin B_{12}	0	Biotin	0
Vitamin D	0	Vitamin E	0	Pantothenic acid	0	Phosphorus	5
Vitamin K	0	Thiamin	6	Iodine	0	Magnesium	2
Riboflavin	2	Niacin	3	Zinc	2	Selenium	0
Chromium	0	Molybdenum	0	Copper	6	Manganese	6

Lycopene	0 mcg
Omega-3 fatty acids	30 mg
Beta carotene	0 mcg
Lutein/zeaxanthin	0 mcg
Alpha carotene	0 mcg

Bruschetta on Toast

INGREDIENTS

2 slices any whole wheat bread, toasted

Olive oil spray

1 cup tomatoes, diced

1/4 cup cucumbers, diced

1 tbsp. onion, diced

1 clove garlic, chopped

Oregano, basil and pepper to taste

PREPARATION

1) Coat the bread lightly with an olive oil spray,
cut into quarters, and toast under a broiler until crispy.

2) Mix the other ingredients together and spray
the mixture with a light coat of olive oil.

3) Spread the mixture on top of the bread.

Note: *This is a very healthy snack – and tasty, too!*

NUTRITION FACTS

Makes 2 servings   *Serving size: $^1/_2$ recipe*

Total calories per serving	110	Total protein	4g
Total carbohydrates	18g	Total fat	3.5g
Total fiber	3g	Saturated fat	0.5g

% DAILY REQUIREMENT

Vitamin A	3	Vitamin C	20	Vitamin B_6	11	Folate	10
Calcium	7	Iron	12	Vitamin B_{12}	0	Biotin	0
Vitamin D	0	Vitamin E	0	Pantothenic acid	3	Phosphorus	8
Vitamin K	8	Thiamin	10	Iodine	0	Magnesium	7
Riboflavin	8	Niacin	10	Zinc	4	Selenium	12
Chromium	0	Molybdenum	0	Copper	8	Manganese	26

Lycopene	3240 mcg
Omega-3 fatty acids	0 mg
Beta carotene	87 mcg
Lutein/zeaxanthin	117 mcg
Alpha carotene	1 mcg

Side Dishes

Butternut Squash

INGREDIENTS

1 lb. butternut squash, peeled and cut into cubes

1 tbsp. extra virgin olive oil

Pinch of salt and pepper

$1/2$ tsp. sage

Cinnamon, to taste

PREPARATION

1) Place squash on a flat pan and coat with olive oil, salt, pepper and sage.

2) Place pan in 450° oven for approximately 20-25 minutes and cook until browned on all sides.

3) Remove from oven and sprinkle squash with cinnamon.

NUTRITION FACTS

Makes 4 servings   *Serving size: ¹/₄ recipe*

Total calories per serving	90	Total protein	2g
Total carbohydrates	16g	Total fat	3.5g
Total fiber	1g	Saturated fat	0g

% DAILY REQUIREMENT

Vitamin A	109	Vitamin C	12	Vitamin B_6	6	Folate	7
Calcium	3	Iron	6	Vitamin B_{12}	0	Biotin	0
Vitamin D	0	Vitamin E	0	Pantothenic acid	3	Phosphorus	2
Vitamin K	5	Thiamin	7	Iodine	0	Magnesium	4
Riboflavin	4	Niacin	4	Zinc	1	Selenium	1
Chromium	0	Molybdenum	0	Copper	3	Manganese	14

Lycopene	0 mcg
Omega-3 fatty acids	60 mg
Beta carotene	2159 mcg
Lutein/zeaxanthin	0 mcg
Alpha carotene	462 mcg

Chunky Fried Asparagus Sticks

INGREDIENTS

1 lb. thin asparagus, tough ends cut off

3/4 cup whole wheat flour

1 egg, beaten with 1 tbsp. water

2 tbsp. extra virgin olive oil

PREPARATION

1) Wash the asparagus; dry and coat with flour.

2) Beat egg with water and pour in dish large enough to hold the asparagus.

3) Dip coated asparagus into the egg to fully coat.

4) In a shallow frying pan, heat the olive oil and cook the asparagus until browned on both sides.

5) Drain excess oil on paper towels and serve while still warm.

NUTRITION FACTS

Makes 4 servings   Serving size: 4 oz.

Total calories per serving	180	Total protein	8g
Total carbohydrates	21g	Total fat	9g
Total fiber	5g	Saturated fat	1.5g

% DAILY REQUIREMENT

Vitamin A	23	Vitamin C	60	Vitamin B_6	11	Folate	58
Calcium	4	Iron	11	Vitamin B_{12}	2	Biotin	0
Vitamin D	1	Vitamin E	0	Pantothenic acid	6	Phosphorus	17
Vitamin K	6	Thiamin	16	Iodine	0	Magnesium	12
Riboflavin	15	Niacin	14	Zinc	10	Selenium	30
Chromium	0	Molybdenum	0	Copper	13	Manganese	54

Lycopene	0 mcg
Omega-3 fatty acids	80 mg
Beta carotene	2 mcg
Lutein/zeaxanthin	86 mcg
Alpha carotene	0 mcg

Marshmallow Covered Sweet Potatoes

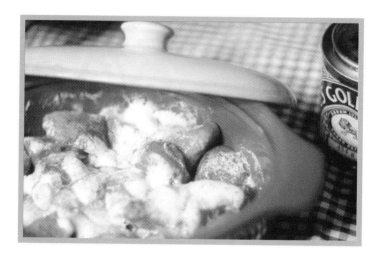

INGREDIENTS

1/4 cup walnuts, chopped

1/4 cup light brown sugar

1 tsp. cinnamon

4 sweet potatoes, peeled, cooked and cut into 1-inch slices

Olive oil spray

1/2 cup mini-marshmallows

PREPARATION

1) Mix the nuts, sugar and cinnamon.

2) Combine mixture with the cooked sweet potatoes, mixing gently.

3) Place in a baking dish and spray with olive oil until lightly coated.

4) Sprinkle marshmallows on top and place in 350° oven
until the marshmallows are melted.

Nutrition Facts

Makes 4 servings   Serving size: ¹/₄ recipe

Total calories per serving	220	Total protein	4g
Total carbohydrates	41g	Total fat	4.5g
Total fiber	4g	Saturated fat	0g

% Daily Requirement

Vitamin A	369	Vitamin C	5	Vitamin B$_6$	16	Folate	4
Calcium	5	Iron	7	Vitamin B$_{12}$	0	Biotin	0
Vitamin D	0	Vitamin E	0	Pantothenic acid	12	Phosphorus	10
Vitamin K	3	Thiamin	8	Iodine	0	Magnesium	13
Riboflavin	7	Niacin	4	Zinc	4	Selenium	3
Chromium	0	Molybdenum	0	Copper	17	Manganese	33

Lycopene	0 mcg
Omega-3 fatty acids	160 mg
Beta carotene	11,063 mcg
Lutein/zeaxanthin	0.7 mcg
Alpha carotene	9 mcg

Creamed Spinach

INGREDIENTS

3 cups fresh or frozen spinach, cooked

1/2 cup onions, chopped into small pieces

1 tsp. olive oil

Salt and pepper, to taste

1/2 package of silken tofu

1/2 cup light soy milk

PREPARATION

1) Drain excess water from spinach.

2) Puree spinach in a blender or food processor until smooth.

3) Sauté onions in oil until soft and add to spinach in blender; add salt, pepper, tofu and soy milk.

4) Blend until smooth.

NUTRITION FACTS

Makes 4 servings   *Serving size: 1 cup*

Total calories per serving   150   Total protein   7g

Total carbohydrates   23g   Total fat   2.5g

Total fiber   3g   Saturated fat   0g

% DAILY REQUIREMENT

Vitamin A	80	Vitamin C	40	Vitamin B_6	2	Folate	1
Calcium	60	Iron	13	Vitamin B_{12}	0	Biotin	0
Vitamin D	0	Vitamin E	0	Pantothenic acid	0	Phosphorus	2
Vitamin K	1	Thiamin	3	Iodine	0	Magnesium	3
Riboflavin	1	Niacin	1	Zinc	1	Selenium	0
Chromium	0	Molybdenum	0	Copper	3	Manganese	1

Lycopene	0 mcg
Omega-3 fatty acids	0 mg
Beta carotene	0.24 mcg
Lutein/zeaxanthin	1 mcg
Alpha carotene	0 mcg

Desserts

Baked Apples and Walnuts

INGREDIENTS

4 baking apples, peeled and cored

1 cup apple juice, unfiltered

1/2 cup walnuts, chopped

1/2 tsp. cinnamon

1 tsp. brown sugar

PREPARATION

1) Place apples in a baking dish and pour the apple juice over them.

2) Place in a 400° oven and cook until soft
(approximately 45-50 minutes).

3) Remove from the oven and let cool.

4) Spread the walnuts onto a cookie sheet and lightly toast at 350°.
(Keep an eye on the walnuts so they do not burn: 10-15 minutes.)

5) Combine the sugar and cinnamon in a small bowl.

6) Grind the toasted walnuts in a blender to a fine consistency.

7) Mix the walnuts, sugar and cinnamon.

8) Cut the apples into halves and sprinkle walnut mixture over them.

NUTRITION FACTS

Makes 4 servings   Serving size: 1 apple

Total calories per serving	240	Total protein	4g
Total carbohydrates	39g	Total fat	10g
Total fiber	6g	Saturated fat	0g

% DAILY REQUIREMENT

Vitamin A	2	Vitamin C	47	Vitamin B$_6$	9	Folate	3
Calcium	3	Iron	6	Vitamin B$_{12}$	0	Biotin	0
Vitamin D	0	Vitamin E	0	Pantothenic acid	4	Phosphorus	10
Vitamin K	6	Thiamin	3	Iodine	0	Magnesium	11
Riboflavin	4	Niacin	1	Zinc	4	Selenium	4
Chromium	0	Molybdenum	0	Copper	14	Manganese	37

Lycopene	0.08 mcg
Omega-3 fatty acids	330 mg
Beta carotene	61 mcg
Lutein/zeaxanthin	64 mcg
Alpha carotene	0 mcg

Pumpkin Pudding

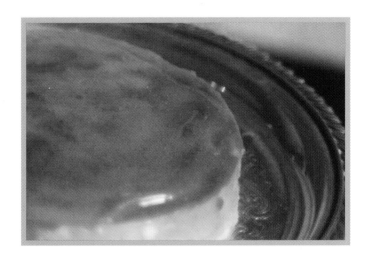

INGREDIENTS

1 15-oz. can puréed pumpkin

1 tsp. cinnamon

$1/2$ cup sugar

2 eggs

$1/2$ tsp. salt

Pinch of nutmeg

12 fluid oz. evaporated skim milk

PREPARATION

1) Mix together all ingredients except the milk until well blended.

2) Add the evaporated milk and pour slowly into the mixture while stirring.

3) Transfer to a glass baking dish and bake at 350° for 40 minutes, or until top is slightly brown.

4) Cool in the refrigerator and serve.

NUTRITION FACTS

Makes 4 servings   Serving size: ¹/₄ recipe

Total calories per serving	240	Total protein	11g
Total carbohydrates	45g	Total fat	2.5g
Total fiber	3g	Saturated fat	1g

% DAILY REQUIREMENT

Vitamin A	341	Vitamin C	9	Vitamin B$_6$	7	Folate	8
Calcium	32	Iron	12	Vitamin B$_{12}$	9	Biotin	0
Vitamin D	21	Vitamin E	0	Pantothenic acid	14	Phosphorus	27
Vitamin K	21	Thiamin	6	Iodine	0	Magnesium	13
Riboflavin	27	Niacin	3	Zinc	9	Selenium	14
Chromium	0	Molybdenum	0	Copper	8	Manganese	9

Lycopene	0 mcg
Omega-3 fatty acids	10 mg
Beta carotene	7132 mcg
Lutein/zeaxanthin	0 mcg
Alpha carotene	4927 mcg

Rice Pudding

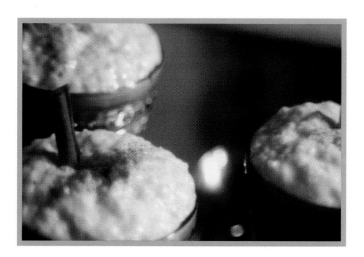

INGREDIENTS

1 package (10 oz.) microwavable organic brown rice
(Trader Joe's brand is good.)

2 eggs

1 cup nonfat vanilla soy milk

$1/2$ tsp. almond extract

$1/4$ cup sugar

2 cinnamon sticks

Cinnamon powder, to taste

PREPARATION

1) Follow the package directions for cooking the rice but deduct 30 seconds
of the recommended cooking time.
Note: *The rice will not be fully cooked at this point.*

2) Beat the eggs in a bowl until thoroughly mixed;
add the soy milk and almond extract.

3) Pour the liquid mixture into a pot and mix in the rice.

4) Add cinnamon sticks and cook on medium heat. Slowly mix in the sugar and cook until rice is soft and the mixture thickens–about 5 -10 minutes.

5) Remove from heat and put mixture into pan or individual serving dishes.

6) Let cool and place in refrigerator.

7) Sprinkle with cinnamon before serving.

Nutrition Facts

Makes 2 servings   *Serving size: ¹/2 cup*

Total calories per serving	210	Total protein	5g
Total carbohydrates	40g	Total fat	2.5g
Total fiber	2g	Saturated fat	0.5g

% Daily Requirement

Vitamin A	4	Vitamin C	0	Vitamin B_6	9	Folate	3
Calcium	7	Iron	5	Vitamin B_{12}	4	Biotin	0
Vitamin D	8	Vitamin E	0	Pantothenic acid	6	Phosphorus	11
Vitamin K	0	Thiamin	8	Iodine	0	Magnesium	11
Riboflavin	6	Niacin	7	Zinc	5	Selenium	8
Chromium	0	Molybdenum	0	Copper	5	Manganese	54

Lycopene	0 mcg
Omega-3 fatty acids	10 mg
Beta carotene	2 mcg
Lutein/zeaxanthin	61mcg
Alpha carotene	0 mcg

Strawberry Shortcake

INGREDIENTS

1 low-fat bran muffin

1/2 cup nonfat vanilla or strawberry yogurt

1 cup strawberries, thinly sliced

PREPARATION

1) Cut the bran muffin in half and spread the yogurt on both halves.

2) Divide the strawberries and place on top of the yogurt.

Note: *This is a healthy dessert everyone can enjoy!*

NUTRITION FACTS

Makes 2 servings   Serving size: 1/2 muffin

Total calories per serving	190	Total protein	5g
Total carbohydrates	40g	Total fat	1.5g
Total fiber	3g	Saturated fat	0g

% DAILY REQUIREMENT

Vitamin A	0	Vitamin C	77	Vitamin B$_6$	2	Folate	5
Calcium	10	Iron	5	Vitamin B$_{12}$	0	Biotin	0
Vitamin D	0	Vitamin E	0	Pantothenic acid	1	Phosphorus	2
Vitamin K	2	Thiamin	6	Iodine	0	Magnesium	2
Riboflavin	6	Niacin	4	Zinc	1	Selenium	0
Chromium	0	Molybdenum	0	Copper	2	Manganese	15

Lycopene	0 mcg
Omega-3 fatty acids	50 mg
Beta carotene	5 mcg
Lutein/zeaxanthin	20 mcg
Alpha carotene	0 mcg

Fruit Salad & Caramel

INGREDIENTS

1 orange, cut into bite-size pieces

1 grapefruit, cut into bite-size pieces

1 banana, cut into thin slices

3 candy caramel pieces

PREPARATION

1) Mix sliced fruit and divide into 3 servings.

2) Melt the caramel in a dish over simmering water. (Be careful not to burn the caramel.)

3) Drizzle the melted caramel over the fruit.

NUTRITION FACTS

Makes 3 servings   *Serving size: 1 cup*

Total calories per serving	130	Total protein	2g
Total carbohydrates	30g	Total fat	1g
Total fiber	3g	Saturated fat	1.5g

% DAILY REQUIREMENT

Vitamin A	25	Vitamin C	100	Vitamin B$_6$	11	Folate	9
Calcium	5	Iron	1	Vitamin B$_{12}$	0	Biotin	0
Vitamin D	0	Vitamin E	0	Pantothenic acid	6	Phosphorus	4
Vitamin K	1	Thiamin	6	Iodine	0	Magnesium	6
Riboflavin	6	Niacin	3	Zinc	1	Selenium	2
Chromium	0	Molybdenum	0	Copper	5	Manganese	7

Lycopene	1256 mcg
Omega-3 fatty acids	20 mg
Beta carotene	621 mcg
Lutein/zeaxanthin	15 mcg
Alpha carotene	14 mcg

Meal Plan Suggestions

BREAKFAST

- 3 egg white omelet
- 2 slices whole wheat toast
- 1 cup skim milk

- 1 cup high-fiber cereal
- 1 cup milk
- 1 cup strawberries

- 1 cup yogurt with 1/2 cup raspberries & 1 tbsp. wheat germ
- 1 cup fresh orange juice

- 2 whole wheat waffles with 1/2 cup fruit
- 1 cup skim milk

- 1 flax meal French toast with 1 cup blueberries
- 1 cup skim milk

- 2 oz. whole wheat bagel with 2 slices low-fat cheese
- 1 cup orange juice

- 1 cup oatmeal with 1/2 cup strawberries
- 1 cup skim milk

SNACK

- 1 cup blueberries

- 2 tbsp. mixed nuts

- 2 tbsp. nuts

- 3 cups air-popped popcorn

- 2 tbsp. nuts

- 2 tbsp. peanut butter with celery

- 1 cup yogurt
- 1/2 cup blueberries

LUNCH

- 2 cups salad with 1 cup chickpeas, 1/2 cup chopped tomato, 1 oz. cheese & 1 tbsp. low-fat Italian dressing

---

- 3 slices turkey on whole wheat bread with lettuce & tomato
- 1 cup skim milk

- 3 oz. chicken salad
- 2 slices whole wheat bread with lettuce & tomato
- 1 cup skim milk

- 1 cup nonfat yogurt with 1/2 cup blueberries, 2 tbsp. nuts & 1 tbsp. toasted wheat germ

---

- 1 slice whole wheat pizza with tomatoes & fresh mozzarella
- 1 apple

- salad in pita bread with turkey
- 1 banana
- 1 cup skim milk

- 3 oz. tuna salad on whole wheat bagel with tomato & lettuce
- 1 apple

Meal Plan Suggestions

SNACK	DINNER	SNACK
• 2 tbsp. mixed nuts	• 4 oz. chicken • 2 cups broccoli •2 cups whole wheat pasta • 1 cup skim milk	• 1 banana
• 1 cup cut-up peppers with 2 tbsp. bleu cheese dressing	• 2 8-inch tacos with 1 1/2 cups pinto beans & 1/4 cup salsa • 1 cup mixed vegetables	• 1 cup frozen yogurt • 1 cup honeydew
• 1 apple	• 2 cups vegetarian chili with 2 cups bulgar • 1 oz. low-fat cheese	• 1 rice cake with 2 tbsp. apple butter
• 1 cup spinach dip with 1 cup baked tortilla chips	• 4 oz. shrimp stir fry with 2 cups mixed vegetables • 1 cup brown rice • 1 cup skim milk	• 1/2 cup strawberries
• 1 serving hummus with 1 baked whole wheat tortilla	• 2 servings shrimp & oranges with pasta • 1 cup skim milk	• 1/2 cup rice pudding
• 1 cup cut-up vegetables with 2 tbsp. low-fat dressing	• 4 oz. grilled salmon with 2 cups mixed vegetables • baked sweet potato • 1 cup skim milk	• 1 baked apple with walnuts
• 1 cup baked tortilla cut into chips with salsa	• 4 1-oz. turkey meatballs • 1 cup whole wheat pasta with sauce • 2 cups broccoli • 1 cup skim milk	• 2 rice cakes with 2 tbsp. peanut butter & jelly

Glossary of Foods

This glossary contains a selected list of commonly eaten foods that are particularly nutrient-dense. Each item includes a brief explanation of why the food is so healthy. New phytonutrients are being discovered in many foods all the time, giving us even more reasons to include them in our diet.

ALMONDS contain more calcium than any other nut. They are a good source of vitamin E and contain protein, magnesium, fiber and the phytonutrients quercetin and kaempferol. Quercetin and kaempferol are the most abundant flavonoids in the diet; they have anticancer, antiviral and anti-allergy properties. Almonds help protect against heart disease and help to maintain bone health.

APPLES contain vitamin C, soluble and insoluble fiber, potassium and quercetin. Apples are good for cleaning teeth and exercising gum tissue. Because they contain fiber they also help with colon health.

ASPARAGUS are low in calories, contain protein, folate, vitamin C, fiber, beta carotene and glutathione. Asparagus help to protect against heart disease, stimulate the immune system and promote colon health.

BANANAS are a carbohydrate-dense fruit that contain potassium, vitamin B_6, vitamin C and folate. They are a favorite fruit among children as well as adults.

BEANS, including lentils and kidney beans, are a low-fat, high-protein legume. They are high in fiber, B vitamins, folate, iron and phytonutrients. Beans help to lower cholesterol and homocysteine levels, reducing risk for heart disease. They also stabilize blood sugar, help relieve constipation and may reduce the risk of some cancers. The soluble fiber in beans is a source of energy that is released slowly into the bloodstream, keeping the blood glucose from rising too high, stabilizing insulin levels and decreasing the risk of type II diabetes and obesity. This sugar stabilizing effect is a major advantage of eating beans.

BLUEBERRIES are loaded with antioxidants and other nutrition boosters, making them a powerhouse for maintaining our health. They contain polyphenols, carotenoids, folate, vitamin C, vitamin E, niacin, riboflavin, manganese, magnesium and the anticancer component ellagic acid. Blueberries contain high quantities of antioxidants from the anthocyanin family, which is what puts the "blue" in blueberry. The anthocyanins are anticancer and antioxidant phytonutrients. Blueberries seem to slow or possibly reverse the effects that aging has on the brain. They reduce the risk of heart disease and also have some antibacterial properties. Blueberries have a fair amount of fiber, which aids in preventing constipation. Blueberries should be on everyone's regular menu; try to have them at least three times a week. You can even carry them for use as a snack.

BOK CHOY contains vitamin C, folate, fiber, calcium, beta carotene, protein and cancer-fighting phytonutrients.

BROCCOLI is a nutrient-dense vegetable that contains vitamin C, folate, beta carotene, potassium, fiber, calcium, vitamin K, lutein, zeaxanthin, coenzyme Q10, flavonoids and the phytonu-trient sulforaphane, which lowers the incidence of lung, colon and stomach cancers.[1] The cancer-fighting nutrients in broccoli make it one of the most powerful foods we can eat. Broccoli also stimulates the immune system, keeps bones strong, reduces the incidence of cataracts and helps keep the heart healthy.

BROWN RICE contains fiber, vitamin E, selenium, niacin, magnesium and vitamin B_6. Brown rice also contains antioxidants, giving it the added benefit of fighting heart disease.

BRUSSELS SPROUTS contain cancer-inhibiting isothiocyanates, vitamin C, folate, potassium, vitamin K and some beta carotene. Brussels sprouts help fight cancer, stimulate the immune system and lower the risk for heart disease.

BUTTERNUT SQUASH contains vitamin C, magnesium, beta carotene, potassium and fiber.

BUTTON MUSHROOMS supply a fair amount of nutritional value for a food that is low in calories. They contain selenium, B vitamins, copper and the newly discovered anticancer nutrients called triterpenoids.

CANTALOUPES are a good source of beta carotene, vitamin C and potassium. They help to keep skin healthy and reduce the risk of heart disease. They also are important for optimal function of the immune system.

CARROTS contain many carotenoids including alpha and beta carotene, lutein and zeaxanthin. Beta carotene maintains night vision, while lutein and zeaxanthin help to prevent cataracts and age-related macular degeneration. Alpha carotene is a potent antioxidant that helps to prevent cancer and heart disease. Carrots contain soluble fiber that helps to reduce cholesterol absorption.

CAULIFLOWER is low in calories and high in nutritional value. It contains vitamin C, fiber, folate and protein. It has the cancer-fighting phyotnutrients sulforophanes. Cauliflower helps to protect against heart disease and stimulates the immune system.

CHERRIES contain vitamin C, beta carotene, anthocyanins, quercetin and pectin. Pectin is a soluble fiber that helps to reduce cholesterol. The anthocyanins give cherries their anticancer and antioxidant properties while quercetin has anticancer,

antioxidant and anti-inflammatory properties.

CHICK PEAS are high in fiber and protein, low in fat, and high in folate and phytonutrients like isoflavones. They help to keep the colon healthy, lower cholesterol (thereby decreasing the risk for heart disease) and reduce hormone-related cancers.

CHICKEN is a high protein food that kids love to eat. The white meat, without the skin is low in fat. Chicken contains some selenium. It is best to eat chicken with vegetables to add nutrients to the meal.

FLAXSEEDS AND FLAX MEAL contain alpha linolenic acid; lignins, the insoluble plant fiber phytoestrogens that may prevent some hormonally related cancers; and potassium. Flaxseeds are the most important plant source of omega-3 fatty acids. They can reduce cholesterol and lower the risk of heart disease. Flaxseeds need to be well chewed or ground up for proper absorption. Sprinkle flax meal on cereal, in yogurt or on ice cream.

GREEN PEAS are low in fat and high in protein and fiber. They contain vitamin C and folate. Green peas will help reduce cholesterol, reduce heart disease, help relieve constipation and reduce the risk of certain cancers.

OATS are a good source of complex carbohydrates, thiamin, selenium, copper, zinc, folate, vitamin E and fiber. Oats will help lower cholesterol and homocystein levels and thereby reduce the risk of heart disease. Eating oats supplies the body with fiber, antioxidants and some cancer-inhibiting phytonutrients. Eat oatmeal for breakfast—try the real stuff, without the sugar and add fresh fruit.

ORANGES contain large quantities of vitamin C; zinc; selenium; fiber; vitamin B_6; folate; and limonene, a potent phytonutreint found in the peel that stimulates our natural detoxification system and stops cancer before it can begin. Oranges are a nutrient-packed fruit that contain many other minerals and vitamins. Vitamin C helps maintain healthy skin and can also help prevent heart disease. Vitamin C also makes it easier to fight off colds. Great for eating; if drinking orange juice, make sure it is fresh and contains the pulp.

PEANUT BUTTER contains nutrients that help new cells to grow and contribute to healthy teeth and bones: vitamin E,

niacin, folate, monounsaturated fats, zinc, manganese, phosphorus, magnesium and fiber. Peanuts supply lots of energy as well as the nutrients needed to extract the energy from the foods we eat. Peanuts are not actually nuts; they are legumes. They contain resveratrol, a phytonutrient also found in the skin of grapes and wine, which is known to help prevent heart disease and is a powerful anticarcinogen.[2] Eat the natural peanut butter with no added sugar.

PINK GRAPEFRUIT contains vitamin C, folate, pectin (a soluble fiber that lowers cholesterol and helps to lower glucose absorption and therefore diminish the rise in insulin after eating), potassium, lycopene and beta carotene. Grapefruit is high in naringin, which has multiple benefits (for more details on the benefits of naringin, see p. 51). Pink grapefruit can lower the risk for stroke, cancer and heart disease.

PUMPKIN is a very nutritious food. Lots of heart-protective alpha and beta carotenoids are found in pumpkin. Pumpkins are high in fiber, vitamins C and E and potassium. The high fiber in pumpkin helps to reduce cholesterol and keep the colon healthy. Pumpkin is rich in carotenoids that help to reduce heart disease and lower the risk for some types of cancers. The rich amount of alpha carotene may slow the aging process.[3]

RASPBERRIES contain fiber, vitamin C and the phytonutrients beta carotene, ellagic acid, catechins and monoterpenes. These phytonutrients help fight cancer and help decrease cholesterol levels.[4]

ROMAINE LETTUCE is low in calories, contains vitamins C and E, folate, fiber and beta carotene. Romaine lettuce helps to reduce blood pressure and also boost the immune system; it is a heart healthy food.

SALMON is rich in omega-3 fatty acids and B vitamins. The list of benefits of omega-3 fatty acids is endless. This fatty acid reduces heart disease and helps keep skin, nails, and hair healthy; it can also reduce the risk of stroke.

SEA BASS is high in protein and low in calories. Sea bass contains selenium, vitamin B_{12}, and omega-3 fatty acids. Omega-3 fatty acids are important in warding off heart disease.

SNAP BEANS, also known as string beans, contain vitamin C, folate, iron and beta carotene. They also contain fiber and some protein.

SPINACH is rich in carotenoids, folate, vitamin K, iron, magnesium, manganese, alpha lipoic acid, lutein, zeaxanthin, coenzyme Q10 and protein. The mineral combination in spinach helps to control blood pressure and acts as a diuretic in getting rid of excess water in the body. It is better to eat cooked spinach than raw spinach because cooking makes the carotenoids easier to absorb. It is also rich in quercetin which inhibits histamine formation, platelet aggregation and tumor growth. Quercetin also acts as an antioxidant, inhibiting cataract formation and LDL oxidation. Spinach is one of the healthiest foods known.

STRAWBERRIES are second only to blueberries in the amount of antioxidants they contain. They are rich in fiber, vitamin C, manganese and ellagic acid. Strawberries help to keep the immune system functioning well, reduce heart disease and may reduce some cancers. Eat them fresh.

SUNFLOWER SEEDS contain folate, vitamin E, B vitamins, copper, magnesium, selenium, protein and phosphorus. These seeds are great for bone health and they also contain powerful antioxidants to protect against heart disease.

SWEET POTATOES are high in beta carotene, vitamin C, lutein, zeaxanthin, fiber, vitamin B_6 and manganese. Sweet potatoes are full of sweet benefits: they have anticancer properties, they help fight off heart disease, they contain the phytonutrients that help protect against degeneration of the eyes and they may slow the aging process.

TOFU contains all the essential amino acids, selenium, calcium, magnesium, fiber, riboflavin, thiamin, folate, and disease-fighting phytoestrogens (isoflavones). It is the only plant that contains complete protein (all essential amino acids), which is essential for growth. Tofu is a cancer-fighting food that can also lower cholesterol and boost the immune system. The benefits of tofu and the soybeans from which it is made are just beginning to be recognized.

TOMATOES contain lycopene, vitamin C, vitamin A, folate, fiber, carotenoids and potassium. Their health benefits include cancer prevention, immune stimulation and prevention of heart disease. Though tomatoes are technically fruits they are usually thought of as vegetables. Tomatoes are the main ingredient in ketchup and tomato sauce, foods that most children consume, making it easy to add them to our daily menu. Tomatoes are in the RED foods category; count them as a fruit or vegetable in the plan.

TURKEY is the leanest of all meats and it is packed with protein. It is an excellent source of B vitamins, phosphorus, selenium, zinc and some iron. Turkey is an animal meat that is actually healthy for the heart.

WALNUTS are a power-packed nut, rich in omega-3 fatty acids (protective against heart attacks) and antioxidants. They also contain plant sterols, ellagic acid, fiber, protein, magnesium, copper and manganese. They can lower blood cholesterol, help to protect against heart disease and may decrease the risk for diabetes. Other power-packed nuts include almonds, pistachios, Brazil nuts, pecans and pumpkin seeds.

WHEAT GERM is a good source of protein, B vitamins, minerals, iron and the fiber that helps to reduce cholesterol. The germ is the inner layer of the wheat berry that is packed with vitamins and phytonutrients. Wheat germ reduces cholesterol and stabilizes glucose. Sprinkle wheat germ on cereal, yogurt or ice cream.

YOGURT is an excellent source of calcium, protein, riboflavin, phosphorus and vitamin B_{12}. Since yogurt contains calcium and phosphorus, it is excellent for bone growth. The lactobacillus in yogurt produces lactic acid in the intestine, which inhibits the growth of pathogenic bacteria. The cell walls of these bacteria stimulate the immune system. It is important to eat yogurt with live bacteria.

Appendix 1

figure 1

Prevalence of overweight among children & adolescents ages 6-19 years

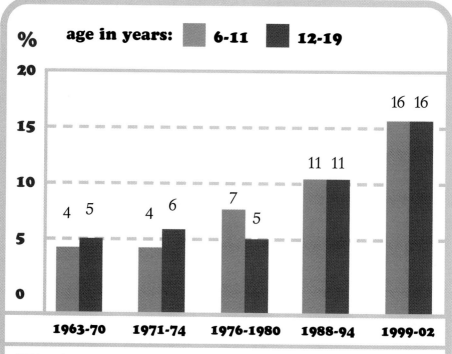

NOTE: Excludes pregnant women starting with 1971-74. Pregnancy status not available for 1963-65 and 1966-1970. Data for 1963-1965 are for children 6-11 years of age; data for 1966-70 are for adolescents 12-17 years of age, not 12-19 years. SOURCE: CDC/NCHS, NHES and NHANES.

Source: Center for Disease Control
http://www.cdc.gov/nchs/products/pubs/pubd/hestats/overwght99.htm

Appendix 2

Quick Facts:
Economic & Health Burden
of Chronic Disease

Disease/ Risk Factors	Morbidity (Illness)	Mortality (Death)	Direct Cost/ Indirect Cost
DIABETES	Over 18.2 million Americans have diabetes, and about one third of them don't know that they have the disease. By 2050, an estimated 29 million U.S. residents are expected to have diagnosed diabetes.	Diabetes is the sixth leading cause of death. Over 200,000 people die each year of diabetes-related complications.	The estimated economic cost of diabetes in 2002 was $132 billion. Of this amount, $92 billion was due to direct medical costs and $40 billion to indirect costs such as lost workdays, restricted activity, and disability due to diabetes.
HEART DISEASE & STROKE	More than 70 million Americans (over one-fourth of the population) live with a cardiovascular disease.	Over 927,000 Americans die of cardiovascular disease or stroke each year, which amounts to one death every 34 seconds.	The cost of cardiovascular disease and stroke in the United States in 2005 is projected to be $394 billion including direct and indirect costs.
CANCER	About 1.4 million new cases of cancer will be diagnosed in 2005 alone. This estimate does not include in situ (preinvasive) cancer or the more than 1 million cases of non-melanoma skin cancer expected to be diagnosed this year.	Cancer is the second leading cause of death in the United States. In 2005, an estimated 570,280 Americans or more than 1,500 people a day, will die of cancer.	NIH estimates that the overall costs for cancer in the year 2004 at 189 billion: of this amount, $69 billion for direct medical costs and more than $120 billion for indirect costs such as lost productivity.
OVERWEIGHT/ OBESITY	Between 1980 and 2000, obesity rates doubled among adults. About 60 million adults, or 30% of the adult population, are now obese. Since 1980, overweight rates have doubled among children and tripled among adolescents. About one in every six children (16.5%)—about 9 million young people—are considered overweight.	The latest study from CDC scientists estimates that about 112,000 deaths are associated with obesity each year in the United States.	Direct health costs attributable to obesity have been estimated at $52 billion in 1995 and $75 billion in 2003. Among children and adolescents, annual hospital costs related to overweight and obesity more than tripled over the past two decades.

Source: Center for Disease Control
http://www.cdc.gov/nccdphp/press/index.htm

Appendix 3

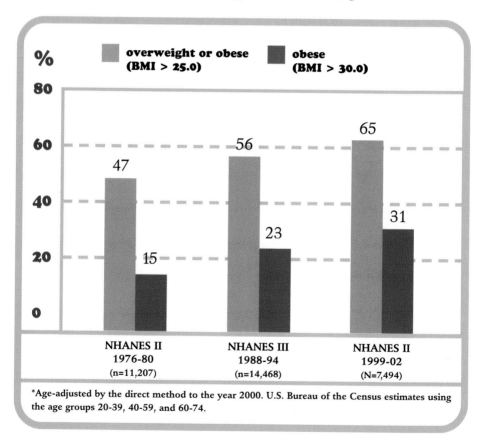

figure 2

Age-adjusted* prevalence of overweight & obesity among U.S. adults, ages 20-74 years

Source: Center for Disease Control
http://www.cdc.gov/nchs/products/pubs/pubd/hestats/overwght99.htm

Appendix 4

Planning a Nutritious Day

This is an easy-to-follow, step-by-step guide to planning your nutrient-filled day

Plan out your grains and nuts for the day.
Adults and adolescents should start with 6 servings of grains
and 1 serving of nuts.
3-4 servings at 3-6 years of age
4-6 servings at age 6- until puberty

Now add fruit into your daily plan:
1^1/$_2$-3 cups for adults and adolescents
1 cup for 3-6 year olds
1^1/$_2$ cups from age 6 until puberty

Next add vegetables to your plan:
2-4 cups for the adults and adolescents
1 cup for 3-6 year olds
1^1/$_2$-2 cups from age 6 until puberty

Continue by adding dairy products to your day:
2-3 servings
Adolescent and adult females need 3-4 servings of dairy/day.

Finally, complete the daily plan by adding
2 small protein servings to the day for adults and adolescents
(1 serving is about the size of a deck of cards)
Children start with 1 protein serving and
increase to 2 servings/day as they grow.

Photocopy this page and use it to help plan your daily nutrition.

Appendix 5

Daily Chart

	FOOD	PORTION SIZE	COLOR GROUP SERVINGS
Breakfast			
Snack			
Lunch			
Snack			
Dinner			
Snack			

Photocopy this page and use it to plan and track your daily nutrition.

Appendix 6

Portion Control: Understanding Serving Sizes for Each Food Category

GRAINS
1 ounce = 1 serving

1 slice of bread	$1/3$ cup of rice
$1/2$ small bagel	$1/2$ cup cooked cereal
$1/2$ cup pasta	1 oz. cold cereal
$1/2$ small bun	$1/2$ pita
$1/2$ large tortilla	3-4 cups air-popped popcorn

FRUIT
1 serving = 1 cup

1 medium sized fruit   8 oz. 100% fruit juice   1 cup fruit

VEGETABLE
1 serving = 1 cup

2 cups RAW leafy vegetables   1 potato (sweet or white)
1 cup cooked vegetables

DAIRY
1 serving

1 cup milk
1 cup yogurt
$1^{1}/2$ oz. hard cheese
1 slice of processed cheese

PROTEIN
1 serving

3 slices of deli meat
4 oz. meat
Cooked meat serving = the size of a deck of cards
$1^{1}/2$ cups beans
3-4 egg whites

References

Foreword

1. National Center for Health Statistics. (n.d.). Prevalence of Overweight Among Children and Adolescents: United States, 1999-2002. Retrieved September 10, 2006 from http://www.cdc.gov/nchs/products/pubs/pubd/hestats/overwght99.htm

Introduction

1. U.S. Dept. of Health and Human Services. Centers for Disease Control and Prevention. (n.d.). Preventing Obesity and Chronic Diseases Through Good Nutrition and Physical Activity. Retrieved September 10, 2006 from http://www.cdc.gov/nccdphp/publications/factsheets/Prevention/obesity.htm

2. U.S. Dept. of Health and Human Services. Centers for Disease Control and Prevention. (2006). Physical Activity and Good Nutrition: Essential Elements to Prevent Chronic Diseases and Obesity. Retrieved September 10, 2006 from http://www.cdc.gov/nccdphp/publications/aag/dnpa.htm

3. World Health Organization. (2006). Facts Related to Chronic Disease. Retrieved September 10, 2006 from http://www.who.int/dietphysicalactivity/publications/facts/chronic/en/index.html

4. Amisola, R.V. B., & Jacobson, M. S. (2003). Physical activity, exercise, and sedentary activity: Relationship to the causes and treatment of obesity. *Adolescent Medicine, 14*(1), 23-25.

5. Miller, J., Rosenbloom, A., & Silverstein, J. (2004). Childhood obesity. *Journal of Clinical Endocrinology and Metabolism, 89*(9), 4211-4218.

Chapter One

1. Gidding, S. S. (1996). Understanding obesity in youth. A statement for healthcare professionals from the Committee on Atherosclerosis and Hypertension in the Young of the Council on Cardiovascular Disease in the Young and the Nutrition Committee, American Heart Association Writing Group. *Circulation, 94*(12), 3383-3387.

2. U.S. Dept. of Health and Human Services. Centers for Disease Control and Prevention. (2006). Physical Activity and Good Nutrition: Essential Elements to Prevent Chronic Diseases and Obesity. Retrieved September 10, 2006 from http://www.cdc.gov/nccdphp/publications/aag/dnpa.htm

3. World Health Organization. (2006). Obesity and Overweight. Retrieved September 10, 2006 from http://www.who.int/dietphysicalactivity/publications/facts/obesity/en/index.html

4. Kris-Etherton, P. M. (2004). Bioactive compounds in nutrition and health-research methodologies for establishing biological function: The antioxidant and anti-inflammatory effects of flavonoids on atherosclerosis. *Annual Review of Nutrition,* 24, 511-538.

5. Borek, C. (2005). Antioxidants and the prevention of hormonally regulated cancer. *Journal of Men's Health & Gender,* 2(3), 346-352.

6. World Health Organization. Facts Related to Chronic Disease. (2006). Retrieved September 10, 2006 from http://www.who.int/dietphysicalactivity/publications/facts/chronic/en/index.html

7. National Center for Health Statistics. (n.d.). Prevalence of Overweight Among Children and Adolescents: United States, 1999-2002. Retrieved September 10, 2006 from http://www.cdc.gov/nchs/products/pubs/pubd/hestats/overwght99.htm

8. Fisher, E. A., Van Horn, L., & McGill, H. C. (1997). Nutrition and children. *Circulation,* 95, 2332-2333.

9. American Academy of Pediatrics, Committee on Sports Medicine and Committee on School Health. (2000). Physical fitness and activity in school. *Pediatrics,* 105(5), 1156-1157.

10. Paluska, S. A. (2002). The role of physical activity in obesity management. *Clinics in Family Practice,* 4(2), 369.

11. Faigenbaum, A. D. (2000). Strength training for children and adolescents. *Clinics in Sports Medicine,* 19(4), 593-615.

12. Sothern, M. S. (1999). Motivating the obese child to move: The role of structured exercise in pediatric weight management. *Southern Medical Journal,* 92(6), 577-584.

13. American Academy of Pediatrics, Committee on Sports Medicine and Fitness. (2001). Strength training by children and adolescents. *Pediatrics,* 107(6), 1470-1472.

Chapter Two

1. Freedman, D. S., Dietz, W. H., Srinivasan, S. R., & Berenson, G. S. (1999). The relation of overweight to cardiovascular risk factors among children and adolescents: The Bogalusa heart study. *Pediatrics,* 103(6), 1175-1182.

2. Davis, P. H. (2001). Carotid intimal-medial thickness is related to cardiovascular risk factors measured from childhood through middle age: The Muscatine study. *Circulation,* 104(23), 2815-2819.

3. Opara, E. C. Antioxidants and micronutrients. (2006). *Disease a Month,* 52(4), 151-63.

4. Bertl, E. (2006). Inhibition of angiogenesis and endothelial cell functions are novel sulforaphane-mediated mechanisms in chemoprevention. *Molecular Cancer Therapeutics, 5*(3), 575-585.

5. Tattelman, E. (2005, July). Health effects of garlic. *American Family Physician, 72*(1), 103-106.

6. Rackley, J. D. (2006). Complementary and alternative medicine for advanced prostate cancer. *Urologic Clinics of North America, 33*(2), 237-246.

7. Ibid.

8. Choi, S. (2005). Bax and Bak are required for apoptosis induction by sulforaphane, a cruciferous vegetable-derived cancer chemopreventive agent. *Cancer Research, 65*(5), 2035-2043.

9. U.S. Dept. of Health and Human Services. Centers for Disease Control and Prevention. (n.d.). Preventing Obesity and Chronic Diseases Through Good Nutrition and Physical Activity. Retrieved September 10, 2006 from http://www.cdc.gov/nccdphp/publications/factsheets/Prevention/obesity.htm

10. Woods, J. A. (2006). Exercise, Inflammation, and Innate Immunity. *Neurologic Clinics, 24*(3), 585-599.

11. Watts, K. (2004). Effects of exercise training on vascular function in obese children. *Journal of Pediatrics, 144*(5), 620-625.

12. U.S. Dept. of Health and Human Services. Centers for Disease Control and Prevention. (2006). Physical Activity and Good Nutrition: Essential Elements to Prevent Chronic Diseases and Obesity. Retrieved September 10, 2006 from http://www.cdc.gov/nccdphp/publications/aag/dnpa.htm

13. World Health Organization. (2006). Facts Related to Chronic Disease. Retrieved September 10, 2006 from http://www.who.int/dietphysicalactivity/publications/facts/chronic/en/index.html

14. Ibid.

15. U.S. Dept. of Health and Human Services. Centers for Disease Control and Prevention. (n.d.). Preventing Obesity and Chronic Diseases Through Good Nutrition and Physical Activity. Retrieved September 10, 2006 from http://www.cdc.gov/nccdphp/publications/factsheets/Prevention/obesity.htm

16. World Health Organization. (2006). Facts Related to Chronic Disease. Retrieved September 10, 2006 from http://www.who.int/dietphysicalactivity/publications/facts/chronic/en/index.html

17. Ibid.

18. U.S. Dept. of Health and Human Services. Centers for Disease Control and Prevention. (n.d.). Preventing Obesity and Chronic Diseases Through Good Nutrition and Physical Activity. Retrieved September 10, 2006 from http://www.cdc.gov/nccdphp/publications/factsheets/Prevention/obesity.htm

Chapter Three

1. Wardle, J. (2003). Increasing children's acceptance of vegetables; a randomized trail of parent-led exposure. *Appetite, 40*(2), 155-162.

2. Fowler-Brown, A., Kahwati, L. C. (2004). Prevention and treatment of overweight in children and adolescents. *American Family Physician, 69*(11), 2591-2598.

3. Katzmarzyk, P. T. (2004). Body Mass Index, waist circumference, and clustering of cardiovascular risk factors in a biracial sample of children and adolescents. *Pediatrics, 114*(2), e198-e205.

4. Bray, G. A. (2005). Beyond energy balance: there is more to obesity than kilocalories. *Journal of the American Dietary Association, 105*(5 Suppl. 1), S17-S23.

5. Makris, A. P. Dietary approaches to the treatment of obesity. (2005). *Psychiatric Clinics of North America, 28*(1), 117-139.

6. Beyer, P. L. (2005). Fructose intake at current levels in the United States may cause gastrointestinal distress in normal adults. *Journal of the American Dietary Association, 105*(10), 1559-1566.

7. Ludwig, D. S. (2002). The glycemic index: Physiological mechanisms relating to obesity, diabetes, and cardiovascular disease. *Journal of the American Medical Association, 287*(18), 2414-2423.

Chapter Four

1. Covington, M. B. Omega-3 fatty acids. (2004). *American Family Physician, 70*(1), 133-140.

2. DeFilippis, A. P. (2006). Understanding omega-3's. *American Heart Journal, 151*(3), 564-570.

3. Kalmijn, S. (2004). Dietary intake of fatty acids and fish in relation to cognitive performance at middle age. *Neurology, 62*(2), 275-280.

4. Mitchell, D. C. (2003). DHA-rich phospholipids optimize G-Protein-coupled signaling. *Journal of Pediatrics, 143*(Suppl. 4), S80-S86.

5. Covington, M. B. Omega-3 fatty acids. (2004). *American Family Physician, 70*(1), 133-140.

6. Thomas, D. R. Vitamins in health and aging. (2004). *Clinics in Geriatric Medicine, 20*(2), 259-274.

7. Kullavanijaya, P. Photoprotection. (2005). *Journal of American Academy of Dermatology, 52*(6), 937-958.

8. Johnston, N. (2004). Sulforaphane halts breast cancer cell growth. *Drug Discovery Today, 9*(21), 908.

9. Frydoonfar, H. R. (2004). Sulforaphane inhibits growth of a colon cancer cell line. *Colorectal Disease, 6*(1), 28-31.

10. Lanzotti, V. (2006). The analysis of onion and garlic. *Journal of Chromatography A, 1112*(1-2), 3-22.

11. Ibid.

12. Ibid.

13. Jung, U. J. (2003). Naringin supplementation lowers plasma lipids and enhances erythrocyte antioxidant enzyme activities in hypercholesterolemic subjects. *Clinical Nutrition, 22*(6), 561-568.

14. Jung, U. J. (2006). Effect of citrus flavonoids on lipid metabolism and glucose-regulating enzyme mRNA levels in type-2 diabetic mice. *International Journal of Biochemistry and Cell Biology, 38*(7), 1134-1145.

15. Jagetia, G. C. (2004). Influence of naringin on ferric iron induced oxidative damage in vitro. *Clinica Chimica Acta, 347*(1-2), 189-197.

16. Fang, C. Y. (2005). Correlates of soy food consumption in women at increased risk for breast cancer. *Journal of the American Dietary Association, 105*(10), 1552-1558.

17. Dewell, A. (2006). Clinical review: A critical evaluation of the role of soy protein and isoflavone supplementation in the control of plasma cholesterol concentrations. *Journal of Clinical Endocrinology and Metabolism, 91*(3), 772-780.

18. Fang, C. Y. (2005). Correlates of soy food consumption in women at increased risk for breast cancer. *Journal of the American Dietary Association, 105*(10), 1552-1558.

19. Ibid.

20. Huang, Y. (2005). Decreased circulating levels of tumor necrosis factor-alpha in postmenopausal women during consumption of soy-containing isoflavones. *Journal of Clinical Endocrinology and Metabolism, 90*(7), 3956-3962.

21. Hsu, S. (2005). Green tea and the skin. *Journal of American Academy of Dermatology, 52*(6), 1049-1059.

22. Sumpio, B. E. (2006). Green tea, the "Asian paradox," and cardiovascular disease. *Journal of the American College of Surgeons, 202*(5), 813-825.

Chapter Seven

1. Mutter, K. L. (2003). Prescribing antioxidants (1st ed.). In D. Rakel (Ed.), *Integrative Medicine* (pp. 735-741). Philadelphia: W.B. Saunders.

Chapter Eight

1. Mattes, R. D. (2005). Appetite: measurement and manipulation misgivings. *Journal of the American Dietary Association, 105*(5 Suppl 1), S87-S97.

Chapter Nine

1. Gaziano, J. M., Manson, J. E., & Ridker, P. M. (2005). Primary and Secondary Prevention of Coronary Heart Disease (7th ed.). In Zipes, *Braunwald's heart disease: A textbook of cardiovascular medicine* (pp. 1057-1074). Philadelphia: W.B. Saunders.

2. Gyr, B. M. (2003). Strength training in children and adolescents (2nd ed.). In DeLee and Drez (Eds.), *Orthopaedic Sports Medicine* (pp. 731-735). Baltimore: W. B. Saunders.

3. Nordstrom, A. (2006). Sustained benefits from previous physical activity on bone mineral density in males. *Journal of Clinical Endocrinology and Metabolism, 91*(7), 2600-2604.

4. Committee on Sports Medicine and Fitness, American Academy of Pediatrics. (2000). Climatic heat stress and the exercising child and adolescent. *Pediatrics 106*(1 Pt 1), 158-159.

Chapter Ten

1. Kaput, J. (2005). Decoding the pyramid: A systems-biological approach to nutrigenomics. *Annals of the New York Academy of Sciences, 1055* (Annals 1323.011), 64–79.

2. Mutch, D. M. (2005). Nutrigenomics and nutrigenetics: The emerging faces of nutrition. *FASEB Journal 19*(12), 1602-1616.

Glossary

1. Johnston, N. (2004). Sulforaphane halts breast cancer cell growth. *Drug Discovery Today, 9*(21), 908.

2. Opara, E. C. Antioxidants and micronutrients. (2006). *Disease a Month, 52*(4), 151-63.

3. Ibid.

4. Ibid.

\